Yoga Sutras of Patanjali

Yoga Sutras of Patanjali

Part One, Pada One
Sutras 1.1 - 1.29

A Commentary

Margo Morris

Saints & Mangoes, Los Angeles, CA, USA

Publisher's Cataloging-in-Publication Data:

Names: Morris, Margo, 1949- author.
Title: Yoga sutras of Patanjali : part one, pada one 1.1-1.29, a commentary / Margo Morris.
Description: Los Angeles : Saints & Mangoes, 2024. | Series: Yoga sutras of Patanjali, pt. 2. | Includes bibliographical references and index.
Identifiers: LCCN 2024906085 (print) | ISBN 979-8-9901952-0-2 (paperback) | ISBN 979-8-9901952-1-9 (hardcover) | ISBN 979-8-9901952-2-6 (ebook)
Subjects: LCSH: Yoga. | Meditation. | Buddhism. | Vedanta. | Sufism. | BISAC: HEALTH & FITNESS / Yoga. | BODY, MIND & SPIRIT / Mindfulness & Meditation. | PHILOSO-PHY / Metaphysics.
Classification: LCC B132.Y6 M34 2024 (print) | LCC B132.Y6 (ebook) | DDC 158.1/3--dc23.

Saints & Mangoes, Los Angeles, CA, USA
saintsandmangoes@gmail.com
saintsandmangoes.com

———— **Preface to Part One, Pada One** ————

This translation and commentary has been in the works for over twenty-five years.

My journey with yoga began in the 1990's, on the island of Maui, where I studied with Gary Kraftsow in the lineage of T.K.V. Desikachar and Tirumalai Krishnamacharya.

From the beginning, it was the yoga sutras that captivated me, and within a few years I had begun to put thoughts on paper. At the time, I felt no real sense of urgency, unlike now.

In the intervening years, I have been busy with life and my spiritual quest has taken place largely in the quiet time around the edges. Perhaps in another time and place I would have been doing my practice in some mountain cave, but in this life my solitary cave was to be found in the midst of the duties my daily life required. Nonetheless, the truth and clarity in the yoga sutras have carried me to a place where I've found some degree of understanding and insight, along with a measure of patience which did not come very naturally.

The teachings of the yoga sutras are an ancient and changeless fountain of guidance, as helpful now as ever. I can honestly say that if this commentary contains any valuable insights, they are the result of the principles and teachings that I embraced and began to apply so long ago.

I sincerely hope that you, dear reader, will find something here that will bring you closer to the fulfillment of your journey.

A supplemental Study Guide to this Commentary is anticipated in 2024.
A Commentary for Part Two, Pada One is scheduled for 2025.

Basic Chanting Guidelines

Chanting the yoga sutras is a time-honored method of connecting to their deepest meaning.

Chanting guides ("svara" marks) are displayed underneath the sutra transliteration on the opening page of each sutra presented herein.

For chanting source materials, including audio aids, the reader may wish to make use of the resources at
saintsandmangoes.com

—— **Basic Chanting Guidelines** ——

Intonation

There are three tones used in chanting the Yoga Sutras.

High note: svarita - vertical line above the letter
Middle note: udâtta - no marking
Low note: anudâtta - horizontal line under the letter

Basic Pronunciation

Short vowels - (unmarked)

a sounds like the u in cut
i as in bit
u as in put or foot
e as in bay
ai as in sigh
o as in hope
au as in sound

Long vowels - horizontal line over the vowel (a, i, u) means it is held twice as long as an unmarked vowel, and the sound of the vowel is also changed. For example:

a as in father
i as in beet
u as in brute

Consonants:

s with any marking above or below becomes "sh"
c is always "ch"
h with under dot is pronounced as echo of previous vowel

──── **Introduction** ────

The incomparable legacy of Patanjali is a compendium of 195 (or 196) sutras known as the yoga sutras. As presented by Patanjali, the sutras appear in four padas (chapters): Samadhi Pada, Sadhana Pada, Vibhuti Pada and Kaivalya Pada.

The first chapter, the Samadhi Pada, is comprised of 51 sutras focusing on the philosophical constructs and basic principles of yoga. This current study covers the first 29 sutras of the Samadhi Pada.

Though Patanjali did not present any divisions within the four chapters, for the purpose of study it may be useful to consider the sutras grouped according to content. The groupings utilized here should be seen as a commentarial viewpoint.

──── **Diacritical Marks** ────

For ease of reading and comprehension, diacritical marks for the Sanskrit transliterations have been used only on the initial presentation of each sutra. Thereafter, all Sanskrit words and names are presented without diacritical marks.

Table Of Contents

Acknowledgments

The author gratefully acknowledges the artistry of Murat Kocyigit and Hande Akcayli of Studio Hoid.

Their generosity in creating book cover and layout design, and the countless hours they devoted to implementation, have been instrumental in bringing this book to publication. It was an act of love that can only be answered with the same.

This work is dedicated to V,
The freest of the free.

Chapter 1, Sutra 1
—— *Offering* ——

Kneel on the banks of this still, deep pond.
Drink shamelessly of its reflections.
Where water meets air,
The image of thine own face appears.
But in the depths, as yet impenetrable,
Lies waiting another more subtle form.
Set thy gaze upon the depths...

- Margo Morris

1.1 atha yogānuśāsanam
chanting guide:

atha yogānuśāsanam

Translations

atha	-	now
yoga	-	1. yoke, link, junction, union 2. samadhi
anusasana	-	instruction, direction

1.1 Now the instruction of yoga.

—— Introductory Remarks ——

This sutra serves as a commencement for the teachings that follow.

atha

In regards to the opening sutra, T.K.V. Desikachar, in his translation and commentary, states:

> "the first word, atha, carries the connotation of a prayer, both for an auspicious beginning and a successful conclusion to the work which follows." [1]

This suggests that a prayer is being invoked not only by Patanjali himself, but by every teacher and every student who throughout history has reiterated this sutra and reflected upon its meaning.

The potency of such an invocation becomes apparent in the context of the oral tradition out of which these sutras evolved and within which they are still being taught today. Through the use of this solemn and sacred prayer, we not only dedicate our own efforts, but participate in the conveyance of its living antiquity.

yoga

There are two possible meanings of yoga. The first, derived from the root yuj, means a link, a joining together, as when yoking an ox to a cart. The second meaning, derived from common usage, is samadhi, which refers to a deep state of meditation or complete concentration. Samadhi may be seen as a particular quality of link with one's object of contemplation.

anusasana

Sasana means instruction. The use of the prefix anu (after) suggests that this is a reiteration of previous teachings, presented in an orderly, methodical fashion. The prefix anu also connotes that "the discipline of yoga is being imparted only after the student has demonstrated his purity in observances of self-discipline and has prepared the ground in which the seed is to be sown." [2]

—— Exploration ——

Yoga is a study of the potentiality of human consciousness. To experience that potentiality is to experience a state of conscious wholeness, a simple but extraordinary state of wholeness which is the birthright of every human being.

The natural yearning for this experience of wholeness is inherent in our nature. It is the impulse which underlies the universal desire for self-actualization. Regardless of who we are or where we are, or in what age we live, underlying all that is this yearning for wholeness. No one has to teach us to feel this urge. It is self-evident that there is some potential within us to be uncovered, explored and brought into manifestation.

When we are young we take this for granted. "What will I become, who will I be?" is the question.

Self-actualization has many faces, as varied in wisdom and maturity as the countless faces which have peered out into this world from some inner mysterious place called self. As children, as soon as we begin to identify how to direct our growth through the choices we make, our basic inherent impulse toward self-actualization is expressing itself in specifics. And from that point onward, our particular individual differences tend to obscure the universals. Our urge for self-actualization, however, is not innately linked to the specific ways we attempt to fulfill the urge.

There are two simultaneous paths for us to tread: one leads to an inwardly directed state of conscious wholeness, the other to an outwardly directed state of individual self-expression. In Buddhist terminology this is the distinction between ultimate reality and relative reality, the supra-personal and the personal.

In the practice of yoga the emphasis is on attention. How we use our attention, how we refine it and how we direct it determines our state of consciousness.

If for a moment we are able to drop our personal history, drop the specific ways in which we have creatively experienced ourselves in relation to our circumstances, we create the opportunity to rediscover our innate yearning for wholeness. By grasping that thread of yearning and following it without distraction, we embark more directly upon the path to its source, the source which relentlessly calls us home.

—— **Further Reflections** ——

From a practical standpoint, perhaps the simplest and most direct way of connecting deeply and personally to this sutra, is to reflect upon our own motivations for our study of yoga and the yoga sutras. Personal intentions, desires, expectations and hopes are born from the fertile soil of each individual's unique point of view. In examining the specifics of our present motivations, we have the opportunity to gain insight into what promotes and what inhibits the actualization of our highest values and most pure longings.

Practice Suggestion:

In preparation for each one of your sutra study sessions, try chanting this first sutra, silently or aloud, with full awareness of its meaning to you personally. This initiatory ritual might be combined with a favorite prayer, a poem, or perhaps the Sanskrit chant in praise of Patanjali. You might compose a short poem or prayer that will express your personal intent in your studies.

It may be useful to consider the following:

1. What do you, as a student of yoga, expect to happen as a result of your yoga study? If you do yoga postures or breathing practices, why do you do them? What long range expectations do you have?

2. When we talk about a state of yoga, what does that mean to you? Does it correlate to any personal experiences?

Take your time in considering these questions. As an aid to self-reflection, it is suggested that you write down your answers. It may then be fruitful to update and compare your answers from time to time.

Sutra - 1

Chapter 1, Sutra 2
—— *Offering* ——

...death will not still the mind, nor argument,
nor hopes of after-death.
This world the battle-ground,
yourself the foe Yourself must master.
Eager the mind to seek,
yet oft astray, causing its own distress...

- Arthur Osborne, extract from "Be Still" [3]

1.2 yogaścittavṛttinirodhaḥ

yogaścittavṛttinirodhaḥ

Translations

yoga	-	1. yoke, link, junction, union 2. samadhi
citta	-	mind, intelligence, mind-field
vritti (here: processes)	-	1. activity, function 2. general usage
nirodha (here: harnessing)	-	1. restraint, confinement enclosure (as by a dam or embankment) 2. sprouting, growing, arising

---

1.2 Yoga is harnessing the processes of the mind.

—— Introductory Remarks ——

This sutra introduces a working definition of yoga. Patanjali defines yoga in terms of the mind and its activities. Yoga is the type and quality of relationship that exists between the mind and the processes in which it is engaged.

yoga

Yoga is an ancient school of wisdom offering profound insights into the nature of spiritual transformation. Within this context, yoga is both means and goal:

As means, yoga is a set of principles and practices aimed at achieving an ever-increasing awareness of the normal processes of the mind.

Ultimately, yoga is a state of consciousness which results when the normal processes of the mind have been harnessed and refined to a point where a radical transformation may occur.

In the context of an ongoing yoga practice to which one is deeply committed, yoga may be so fruitful that the distinction between means and goal becomes less apparent.

citta

To get a full sense of the significance of "citta vritti nirodha", it is important to understand that the word citta connotes more than what we normally call "mind". Citta is akin to the totality of the non-physical manifestations of the personality. Citta thus includes thoughts, feelings, emotions, the sense of "I-am-ness", and the deep levels of memory which carry all these forward.

vritti

The vrittis of the citta are the processes or activities with which the citta is occupied. This refers to every aspect of how we normally use our minds and how we normally interact with our objects of perception. It is the act of perception itself which initiates the citta vritti.

nirodha

Ni is a prefix indicating down, back, in, into, within. The word rodha has two main streams of meaning, both of which should be considered:

1. restraint, confinement, enclosure (as by a dam or embankment)

2. sprouting, growing, arising (as a natural development)

—— Exploration ——

As the citta comes into contact with its objects of perception, it is affected by the interaction. This is the normal activity to which the perceiving mind is habituated. But behind this normal process lies a "supranormal" state of consciousness which remains unmodified by the mind or the activities of the mind.

Traditionally, nirodha has been defined as suppression, obstruction, restraint, or alternatively as cessation. All these definitions are technically applicable since we are viewing yoga as both means (suppression, obstruction, restraint) and ultimate goal (cessation).

Yoga exists as a continuum which encompasses the simplest efforts of the neophyte as well as the liberated state of the spiritual master.

The meaning of nirodha is elucidated by the images which emerge from its derivation. A dam or embankment contains, controls and directs the enormous power of a river by virtue of being in equilibrium with the river. Whether the embankment exists naturally or is carefully constructed, it performs effectively only when it possesses the necessary strength and resilience. We might say that a good embankment cradles a river, harnessing its power and delivering it to its destination.

Another useful image comes from the second meaning of rodha which, when combined with ni, suggests the image of a sprouting seed whose normal process of outward and upward growth is turned back toward some innate inner potential.

The notion of controlling the processes of the mind presents difficulties, and one's first grasp of the concept will likely undergo considerable change during an ongoing process of personal development.

One common pitfall is to conclude that meditation is a rigid or lax condition of the mind. Yogic meditation may also be misrepresented as a kind of trance or stupor. Such misunderstandings result in an attempt to negate the mind rather than harness it. A similar confusion revolves around the concept of "emptiness" in Buddhism, where "emptiness" is thought to refer to a vacuum. The missed point is that "emptiness" is empty only of the artifacts and objects of time and space. When these are no longer the primary objects of attention, the mind may rest in the fullness of that which surpasses time and space.

The mind is a tool, a tool capable of perceiving and organizing its perceptions with so much precision that we are continually graced by an awesome communion with the world in which we live. The mind, when used well by the intelligence it serves, is what makes possible the enlightened wisdom of philosophy and religion, as well as the marvels of timeless art and the great discoveries of science and medicine. But the tool comes to us in an imperfect state.

Whether focused on personality or spirituality, the development of the mind requires discipline, determination, some knowledge of what is possible, and a good measure of trust and faith. It takes work to use the mind to its full potential, just as it takes work to use any instrument well. If I sit down to play a Steinway piano and am disappointed with the sounds that emerge, chances are it is not the fault of the Steinway.

———— Further Reflections ————

Yoga is about spiritual transformation. It is about a path of consciously chosen growth, requiring that we redefine ourselves and the reality in which we live. It is about an attempt to touch some sensed but hidden part of ourselves, to come in contact with a Self which carries a mark of true authenticity. This Self lies not outside of us, but inside. It is an inherent part of our nature as human beings.

In spiritual transformation, what exactly is transformed? It is our personalities, meaning our entire complex sense of ourselves and our role in the world: our desires, thoughts, emotions, what we know and what we hope to know, what we do and what we hope to do.

Spiritual transformation does not mean that our personalities become great and powerful. Quite the opposite. The process of spiritual transformation is more a letting go. It is a process which demands a profound humbling of the personal self and a gradual relinquishment of the personal ego as center of one's universe. As for the meaning of spirituality, perhaps that is best left for each of us to carve, with or without the help of a Carver, out of the substance of our own being.

In the words of Tirumalai Krishnamacharya:

Your lord or mine, it does not matter
What matters is, meditate with humility
The Lord, pleased, gives what you seek
And happily will give more.

- Sloka 13, Yoganjalisaram [4]

Sutra - 2

Chapter 1, Sutra 3
—— *Offering* ——

I ride the currents of the wind like an eagle,
And with an eagle's eye, see my brother's feet
Pressing into the shifting contours
Of the terrain below.
Tell me please, my friend, who am I?

I stumble. I fall. Unable to see the path ahead,
I cry out, but find no solace.
What once gave comfort abandons me now.
Alone, beneath a too open sky.
Tell me please, my friend, who am I?

Face to face and heart to heart,
I look into the eyes of my brother.
Beyond the veils of triumph and loss we meet,
And meeting, lose sight of ourselves.
Tell me please, my friend, who am I?

- Margo Morris

1.3 tadā draṣṭuḥ svarūpe 'vasthānam

taḏā draṣṭuḥ svaṟūpe'vasthānam

Translations

tada	-	then
drastuh (here: seer)	-	one who sees
from dris:	-	1. to see, behold, consider 2. to be manifested 3. to appear, become visible
sva	-	own, one's own
rupa	-	form
avasthanam (here: established)	-	1. abiding, residing 2. taking up one's place 3. stability

1.3 Then the seer is established in its own form.

—— Introductory Remarks ——

This sutra explains what occurs in yoga when the citta vritti are successfully harnessed. Then, Patanjali indicates, the seer is established in its self-nature. Standing free of the mitigating influences of the citta vritti, the seer abides in its own place.

tada

Tada references the previous sutra.

drastu

The "seer" refers to the Self or "purusa" of Eastern thought and the Spiritual Man of Western tradition. The seer is the eternal essence of being which is at the core of our human existence. Its nature is pure awareness.

Verbal descriptions of the seer are problematic; it should be remembered that words can only point the way. According to yoga philosophy, the seer, though manifesting within the body-mind complex of the individual, is viewed as being ultimately distinct from this manifestation.

svarupa

The literal meaning of this term is self-form or own-form. Svarupa indicates a form that is authentic or true to its own essential nature, as opposed to a form that merely resembles or is similar (sarupya).

avasthanam

The words "svarupe avasthanam" (established in its ownform), indicate that when the processes of the mind have been successfully harnessed, the seer abides in its own-form (pure awareness). Pure awareness then remains unobstructed by the manifest form of the body-mind.

A Perspective from Buddhist Tradition

The nature of consciousness, or awareness - shepa in Tibetan - is such that it is not at all material... there seems to be an agent "I" who engages in the activity of knowing or being aware; but what we mean by consciousness is that capacity in dependence upon which one knows or is aware. It is, in other words, the activity or process of knowing itself, and as such, it is "mere awareness" or "luminous consciousness". [5]

- H.H. The Dalai Lama

—— Exploration ——

Perhaps the greatest difficulties which arise in the study of this sutra result from the tendency to ascribe the totality of our experiential awareness to purusa, the seer, whereas it is precisely our lack of ability to discriminate between the pure awareness of the seer and the content of our experiential awareness which is being addressed in these sutras. In fact, the study of yoga as a whole is directed towards the challenge of developing the ability to make this distinction.

Our experiential awareness is a function of the pure and unchanging awareness at our core, but is linked to the constantly changing relative reality in which we find ourselves.

As a case in point, yoga philosophy tells us that the seer is always established in its own-form and never has been, or ever could be, separated from itself. Yet as persons who live within time and space, the truth of our experience sometimes encompasses a fundamental and profound sense of separation. Within the field of our experience, and from the standpoint of the attention of our minds, the experience of separation from our essence of being, and the consequent suffering, is a real one.

The mind is like a lens, and awareness is like light passing through a lens. Depending upon the shape of the lens, the light is either concentrated or dispersed. And depending upon any imperfections in the lens, the essential pattern of the passing light is either distorted or remains unaffected.

—— Further Reflections ——

Who am I? What am I?

Spoken or unspoken, whether finding expression through the spontaneous curiosity of a child or emerging in full maturity out of profound insight and desire for truth, these questions have probably arisen in the consciousness of every human being who has tasted that most awesome quality of being human: the experience of BEING a reflectively self- conscious being.

The history of our species is a vibrant and passionate, even if violent, record of self-discovery and self-disclosure.

From the most sublime to the most hideous legacies of our collective journey, what seems to be the one overwhelming, persistent driving force which moves us, is the need to find the defining limits of "me".

What a paradox that I can only find out what I am, by finding out what I am not.

What a gift that I am allowed infinite mistakes along the way.

May I learn to learn with more grace and less harm.

Chapter 1, Sutra 4
—— Offering ——

*...Like a deep truth inside a lie, like the taste of
butter in buttermilk, that's how Spirit is held
in form. For a long time butter stays invisibly
present in the churn mixture...*

- Jalal Al-din Rumi, extract from The Churn" [6]

1.4 vṛttisārūpyamitaratra

vṛttisārūpyamitar<u>a</u>tra

Translations

vritti   -   see 1.2
(here: processes (of the mind))

sarupya   -   1. having the same shape or form
(here: conformity)   2. identity of appearance
                          3. similarity, resemblance

itaratra   -   otherwise, the other (of two)

1.4 Otherwise, conformity with the processes.

—— Introductory Remarks ——

This sutra states that in the absence of harnessing the activities of the mind, the seer (awareness) is in conformity with the processes of the mind, taking the shape of or following the form of its instrument of seeing. Any object is thus perceived through the distortions of the mind, veiling the object's essential nature.

vritti

Traditionally, the vrittis are spoken of in many different ways. Sometimes they are equated to purely mental aspects of perception and cognition. Sometimes they are equated to the mind's ever changing flow of psycho-emotional states such as agitation or tranquility, happiness or sadness, desire or aloofness, distractedness or one-pointedness. In this context, the citta vritti are taken to include all activities of mind.

sarupya

Sarupya stands in contrast to svarupa as described in the previous sutra. Whereas svarupa represents the own-form, the "true form" of the seer, sarupya represents a form that merely resembles svarupa. Interestingly, in Sanskrit drama sarupya refers to a mistaken identity caused by the mutual resemblance of two persons.

Sarupya is often translated as "identification with", meaning that there is an identification of the seer with the processes of the mind. Hoping to minimize the tendency to ascribe actions to the seer, even such a subtle action as identification, sarupya is translated here as conformity. This is intended to connote more a default mechanism than an active process.

Since the seer is permanent, unchanging and formless, what does it mean to say that the seer conforms to the form of the vrittis? It simply means that no distinction is being made between the awareness which underlies all perception, and the complex processes of the mind in relation to that perception.

When the awareness of the seer conforms to the vrittis, we might say that perception is "blinded by appearances" [7], resulting in a misidentification that affects even one's self-perception.

From this comes about a false sense of self, a sense of "I Am" that is linked to the movements of the mind. Once this false sense of self takes hold through continuous activation, it becomes the attitudinal ground from which all perception occurs. It then represents a formidable obstacle to authentic self-perception.

itaratra

The meaning of itaratra is otherwise, indicating what takes place when the processes of the mind have not been harnessed.

A Perspective from Buddhist Tradition

We could say that we only experience consciousness as colored by the object; the perception is almost inseparable from the object....whether we are thinking conceptually or simply having a sensory experience, awareness itself arises with the form or appearance of an object, and as a result, we usually do not recognize it as "mere awareness" or "clear, luminous cognizance". In short, in our ordinary experience, consciousness becomes caught up with the dualistic appearances of "object" and "subject". [8]

- H.H. The Dalai Lama

—— Exploration ——

There are many terms which may be used to express svarupa, the seer. Terms that are common in spiritual traditions include true form, inherent nature, spiritual man, innate man, primary essence, and eternal nature. All of these point to that transcendent part of our being which is independent of our physical form.

In distinguishing between svarupa and sarupya, we should consider drawing both ultimate and relative distinctions. At the ultimate level, once there is no longer any misidentification, the consciousness remains centered unwaveringly in the seer. But short of conditions and circumstances which allow for such a stable state of actualization, for the most part we learn to develop our ability to distinguish between svarupa and sarupya in a relative manner, gradually and successively.

When svarupa is in conformity with the vrittis, it is not only self-perception that is affected. All perception is affected. And that is where our work begins.

Through the field of our everyday perceptions we have the ability to investigate the functioning of our own mental processes. By bringing awareness to the distinctive ways our minds function, for better and for worse, we may in time gain the clarity and understanding needed to find our way home.

Chapter 1, Sutra 5
—— Offering ——

Who am I,
standing in the midst of this
thought-traffic?

- Jalal Al-din Rumi, from The Well" [9]

1.5 vṛttayaḥ pañcatayyaḥ kliṣṭākliṣṭāḥ

vṛttayaḥ pañcatayyaḥ kliṣṭākliṣṭāḥ

Translations

vrttaya	-	processes of the mind (plural of vritti)
pancatayya	-	having five parts, five-fold
klista (here: afflicted)	-	1. afflicted, distressed 2. accompanied by pain and suffering
aklista (here: unafflicted)	-	1. (opp. of klista) non-afflicted 2. not accompanied by pain and suffering

1.5 The processes of the mind are of five categories and are either accompanied or unaccompanied by the klesas.

—— Introductory Remarks ——

This sutra introduces a more in-depth look at the vrittis. Patanjali states that the processes of the mind are of five categories (see sutras 1.6 through 1.11).

vrttaya

Vrttaya is the plural form of vritti.

pancatayya

Panca, meaning five-fold, is derived from pac: to spread out (one's hand), to make clear or evident.

klista -aklista

Klista and aklista are derived from the word klesa. Without making this connection, klista-aklista is deprived of proper context.

Klesa is an umbrella term in yoga philosophy referring to the five root causes of suffering, which may or may not accompany each of the five vrittis:

1. avidya (ignorance of truth)
2. asmita (egoism, I-am-ness)
3. raga (attachment)
4. dvesa (aversion)
5. abhinivesa (longing for immortality).

Avidya is the wellspring of the other four causes of suffering. It is defined as ignorance, but refers specifically to the most fundamental of human ignorances: ignorance of what it truly means to be human.

We all face the false sense of self arising from lack of distinction between the mental processes of our own minds and the perceiving awareness underlying those processes. The mind confuses its own activities with the fundamental awareness of the seer, thinking: "I, the mind, am the seer." Out of this fundamental misperception grows all suffering. When the mind is fully in the grips of "I am the seer", its activities will sooner or later demonstrate as suffering.

Asmita is defined as egoism. It points to the core condition of an individual human being who sees himself as the center of his own universe. At the deepest and most subtle level this egoism may be seen as attributable to the limitation of the experience of I-am-ness, a subject which Patanjali explores in depth in forthcoming sutras.

Raga is defined as attachment or desire. It functions along the lines of "I need power, wealth, beauty, fame..."

Dvesa is aversion. It is the polar opposite of raga and may appear when raga has temporarily expended itself, or when great attachments reverse to become great aversions.

Abhinivesa is the last klesa. It is perhaps the most subtle form of both raga and dvesa. It is that extreme attachment to life which causes an individual to abhor the fact that death is inevitable for living beings.

—— **Exploration** ——

Indian philosophy, like all philosophical systems, loves to make lists. Everything is categorized. As we explore the categories Patanjali has presented, we shall diverge as needed from the more traditional discussions, as our purpose in this study is to gain insight and reflect on how we might hasten our own spiritual growth.

The five categories of citta vritti as described in the next six sutras will be seen to relate specifically to the cognitive functions of mind. Klista aklista, on the other hand, relates to the emotions and attitudes which color an individual's cognition.

Cognition and emotions do not operate independently but in concert. The clarity of each affects the clarity of the other.

Cognition and Quality of Perception

The most basic cognitive activity of the mind is the formation of mental semblances or approximations of perceived objects, based upon thought processes and input from the primary sense organs.

In the process of cognition, the mind sifts through data perceived, selects the data it considers to be most essential based upon its conditioning, and forms the selected data into an approximation of the object perceived.

The degree of correspondence between the mental semblance of an object and the object's actual nature is the comparative measure of quality of perception. The very concept of objectivity derives from this method of comparatively measuring accuracy of perception.

In making objective comparisons we may rely on our own ability to ascertain the object's actual nature through repeated observations, or we may rely on some other authority such as a measuring device, a teacher, an expert, or some generally accepted consensus in regards to the object's actual nature.

Emotional Aspects of the Mind

Emotions, unlike cognition, do not measure the characteristics of an object.

Emotions measure the meaning that an object and its characteristics have for us personally. Thus, when dealing with emotions, we are one step removed from the possibility of assessing appropriate correlations between our experiences and the actual objects and events we are experiencing.

Our emotional mechanisms relate us to our world and allow us to assess the relevance of objects and events to our own needs and interests. Through our emotions we give our perceived objects a certain designated value, even though we often do this unconsciously.

Over time we develop a system of values through which our perceptions are filtered and monitored. In this way our emotions profoundly impact the data selection patterns which we develop within our basic perceptual mechanisms, affecting both current and remembered perceptions.

This can be problematic, for the field of emotions is inherently subjective and we often do not have adequate means of appraising the appropriateness of emotions. Unfortunately, we may remain unaware of our lack of alignment and the profoundness of the filtering effect which that has upon all subsequent perceptions.

In regards to societal values, every society has established norms for what is considered to be acceptable or worthy. At the highest level these social norms represent ideals such as fairness, love, understanding and compassion. Most modern cultures utilize ideals such as these to measure an individual's level of emotional maturity.

In fact we might say that in the realm of subjective emotions, we maintain objectivity through comparison to an ideal, in much the same manner that we check the accuracy of perceptions through comparison with an object's actual characteristics.

Our highest social ideals demonstrate through our emotional and feeling nature. Yet, as each one of us must learn, manifesting love and compassion in the face of difficulties requires a great deal of self-control, often hard-won over a lifetime of effort.

Until the everyday flux of our emotions undergoes the same kind of spiritual transformation as the mental nature, the motility of the emotions serves to obstruct the realization of our highest ideals.

—— Further Reflections ——

This sutra serves as a reminder that our normal object-oriented cognition is accompanied by subjective experience. Simultaneously with our perceptions, we are aware of the value we place upon the objects we perceive. But we are also, at least subliminally, aware of ourselves in the act of perceiving.

This co-existing awareness of both object and subject is a natural characteristic of the self-conscious human being. It may be possible, however, through a process of refinement and purification, to transform the very nature of this subject-object awareness.

As we move deeper into our exploration of the vrittis, we will be able to look practically at our own personal manifestations of the citta vritti. Hopefully, through our study and through our commitment, through our practice and our faith in the possibility for transformation, we will come to a better understanding of how mastery of the vrittis uncovers our higher potentials as human beings.

Chapter 1, Sutra 6
—— *Offering* ——

The gold of your intelligence is scattered
over many clippings and bits of wanting.
Bring them all together in one place...
...grain by grain, collect the pieces.

- Jalal Al-din Rumi, extract from "Masnavi" [10]

1.6 pramāṇaviparyayavikalpanidrāsmṛtayaḥ

pramāṇaviparyayavikalpanidrāsmṛtayaḥ

Translations

pramana (here: correct perception)	-	1. certain knowledge; authority 2. means of acquiring right knowledge
viparyaya (here: misperception)	-	1. reversed, inverted, opposite of 2. mistaking anything to be the reverse or opposite of what it is
from vi:	-	apart, asunder, in different directions

(Continued)

+ paryaya:	-	1. revolution (periodic)
		2. contrariety, opposition
		3. deviation from customary observances
vikalpa (here: imagination)	-	1. imagination, fancy, false notion 2. logic, ideation 3. indecision, irresolution, doubt, hesitation
nidra (here: dreamless sleep)	-	sleep, slumber, sloth
smrtaya (smriti) -		memory, reminiscence

1.6 The five processes of the mind are correct perception, misperception, imagination, dreamless sleep and memory.

—— Introductory Remarks ——

This sutra enumerates the five categories of vritti. According to T.K.V. Desikachar, the five categories of vritti are "interrelated and complex so that each one, except perhaps sleep, should be considered as a matrix or genus of activity rather than a distinct entity with exclusive and limited characteristics." [11]

pramana

In Indian philosophy pramana refers to certain knowledge or the means of acquiring certain knowledge. Pramana is translated here as correct perception.

viparyaya

Viparyaya is translated here as misperception, the opposite of pramana. Paryaya is derived from pari (around) + i (to go), and thus has a connotation of revolving, as a planet revolves, and the resultant alterations in time and space. When coupled with the prefix vi, this suggests the interesting image of spinning or revolving in different directions, implying a lack of coordination or synchronization.

vikalpa

Vikalpa is translated here as imagination; other common translations are fantasy and illusion. Vikalpa is the mental simulation of objects during either a waking or dreaming state and is neither correct perception nor incorrect perception.

nidra

Nidra is usually translated as deep sleep or dreamless sleep, thereby excluding the activity of dreaming. When nidra occurs, the other vrittis are temporarily subdued. Dreaming continues to occur in cyclic alternation with nidra during the sleep cycle, but the two do not occur simultaneously.

smriti

Smriti is translated as memory. Memory is recall of previously acquired knowledge formed under the influence of the other vrittis.

—— **Exploration** ——

Indian philosophy is grounded in epistemology, the study of knowledge, the means of acquiring knowledge, and the question of what constitutes valid authority. Authority is crucial in Indian thought due to its profound reliance on sacred scripture and the tradition of verbal transmission.

This discussion is more focused on an individual's direct relationship to knowledge and how to go about developing and refining one's own authority of mind.

In sutra 1.5 we looked briefly at the way the mind forms sense-images in response to perception. In this sutra we are considering the relationship between the actual characteristics of perceived objects and the images formed by the mind in the act of perception.

Correct perception occurs when there is sufficient correspondence between an actual object of perception and the sense-image of the object formed by the mind.

Misperception occurs when there is insufficient correspondence between an actual object of perception and the sense-image of the object formed by the mind.

Imagination occurs when there is no object with which to compare the images formed by the mind.

The vritti of dreamless sleep occurs when the other four vrittis, along with external sense perception, are temporarily subdued or suspended during the physiological state of sleep.

Memory occurs when images formed by the mind under the influence of the other vrittis are retained and then accessed again at a later time. When we remember something we are dealing with an amalgam of prior and current sense-images and conceptual images. The actual object is either no longer present or not present in the same state. Recalled sense-images do not necessarily correspond exactly to those which were formed at the time of initial perception; they are susceptible to conditions of the mind at the time of recall.

We naturally perceive in "clusters" of information. Through investigating the nature of these "clusters" and the laws which govern them, we may be able to arrive at a better understanding of both ourselves and our universe. And since our minds will, by nature, differentiate, organize and categorize, if we are able to bring our conscious awareness and insight to this process, we are in a better position to enhance the direction of our own personal evolution.

It behooves us to try to define our categories in a way that will aid our clarity and understanding. The idea is not to become so enamored of our own mental activities and knowledge that we lose sight of our intent. In this regard, a well-known science writer humorously points out:

> "Categories are useful only if they mesh with the way the world works...organization for its own sake is useless. I have a compulsive friend whose wife tells callers that he cannot come to the phone because he is alphabetizing his shirts." [12]

In yoga, our purpose is to comprehend the nature of the mind so that ultimately we may purify its contents. Let us be mindful of that intention.

Chapter 1, Sutra 7
—— *Offering* ——

...develop an eye that can see into the Sun.
The world is nailed shut in night,
Waiting for the Sun to come up.
And here it is, hidden in a speck of dirt!

- Jalal Al-din Rumi [13]

1.7 pratyakṣānumānāgamāḥ pramāṇāni

praṭyakṣānumānāgamāḥ pramāṇāni

Translations

pratyaksa	-	direct perception, sense perception
anumana	-	inference
agama (here: authoritative testimony)	-	1. a traditional doctrine or precept 2. anything handed down and fixed by tradition 3. testimony; reliable authority
pramana	-	correct perception

1.7 Direct perception, inference, and authoritative testimony (are the means of) correct perception.

—— Introductory Remarks ——

This sutra presents a working analysis of pramana. The indication is that correct perception may be arrived at through three basic means:

1. direct perception
2. logical inference, combined with one or both of the other two means
3. reliance upon the testimony of an accepted authority

pratyaksa

Pratyaksa is direct perception. It is direct and immediate contact with an object, providing the vivid experience which is the hallmark of direct sensory perception. In pratyaksa the detail is available for scrutiny as long as contact between an object and the senses is sustained.

Direct perception is not a guarantee that perception will be accurate. Nevertheless, the availability of the object offers an optimal opportunity, and conclusions drawn from direct perception may be the most easily verified.

Traditionally, pratyaksa has been associated with the five physical senses, not with intuition or extrasensory perception. The problem with considering extra-sensory perception as means of pramana is establishing appropriate criteria through which accuracy may be determined. If these potentials become more generally actualized, we might also develop the needed criteria for verification.

anumana

The traditional meaning of anumana describes the relation between particulars and universals. It is an analytical reasoning process applied to direct perception. The modern equivalent is inference, which includes both deductive and inductive logic.

The accuracy of conclusions drawn through anumana rests on the accuracy of the original direct perception, accuracy of memory, accuracy of the logical premises applied, and in the case of anumana applied to agama, the accuracy of transmission and reception between the original perceiver and the secondary perceiver.

Some traditional examples of inference:
1. From the presence of smoke, the presence of fire.
2. From the presence of the cat or mouse, the absence of the other.
3. Knowing the sound of one's motor, the arrival of one's car.

In the first example it is safe to infer from the presence of smoke that there is, or has been, the presence of some form of fire. But inferring from the presence of the cat or mouse the absence of the other may be erroneous, as many an uninterested cat will demonstrate. The reliability of the third example depends upon many factors, among them: the actual present condition of one's hearing, the focus or distractedness of one's attention, and the uniqueness of one's motor car.

agama

Agama is translated here as authoritative testimony. Traditionally agama refers to that knowledge which is handed down through spiritual tradition. The essential intent of a genuine spiritual lineage is to preserve and guarantee the continued integrity of agama.

pramana

Pramana is taken here in a relative rather than ultimate sense, drawing a distinction between the perception that occurs in a normal state and that which occurs in a transformational state which uniquely reveals the true essential nature of an object.

A Perspective from Buddhist Tradition

"In Buddhism we speak of three types of phenomena: First, there are evident phenomena that are perceived directly. Second, there are slightly hidden phenomena, which are not accessible to immediate perception... (which) can be known indirectly by inference. Third, there are very concealed phenomena, which cannot be known by either of the two preceding methods. They can be known only by relying upon testimony of someone such as the Buddha.." [14]

- H.H. The Dalai Lama

—— Exploration ——

As we saw in sutra 1.5, each of the five vrittis may be accompanied by the klesas (the causes of suffering) wherein the klista commingle with the aklista.

The processes of the mind which are klista serve to perpetuate the stream of relative reality, which is the arena of the personality, the normal activities of the mind, ordinary everyday consciousness.

Those processes of the mind which are aklista enhance the

dissolution of the klesas and an attenuation of identification with the processes of the mind. They lead in the direction of ultimate reality, the province of the Seer, that indefinable core of pure awareness which is the core essence of human consciousness.

From the standpoint of relative reality, truth is an evolving proposition. We know that our senses do not always provide us with perfect information. We also know that how we interpret what we perceive is colored by many factors.

It is easy to be wrong. The irony about knowing how easy it is to be wrong is the double jeopardy it puts us in. We may end up with a lack of confidence, as confidence is an issue of trust and trust in anything is earned over time.

Lack of confidence in the basic functions of one's mind may manifest in various ways: as self-doubt, timidity, procrastination or indecisiveness. There is also the issue of bluster. Because we learn largely by mimicking those around us, our quest for confidence may produce a fair amount of bluster rather than true confidence.

How can we deal with such paradoxes? How can we balance our need for confidence in ourselves and in our minds, while still recognizing the mind's enormous capacity for distortion and error?

We may start with a realistic evaluation of the capacities of the mind, for it is in fact a very imperfect measuring instrument that gives very different results at different times. This might help us to overturn our emotional identification with being right or wrong. With knowledge of our own fallibility comes a certain ease, as there is not so much at stake in any given circumstance.

We must also recognize that the mind is an enigmatic tool in that it is capable of procuring as much useful information about its own workings as about the objects it is ostensibly measuring.

Realizing this opens up the possibility of reshaping the tool itself, transforming the very nature of mind into something more reliable through a process of purification and refinement.

———— Further Reflections ————

It may be useful to examine cultural factors that influence the meaning of "spiritual authority". It is quite possible that in the pursuit of an in-depth understanding of Eastern spiritual traditions, the issue of what constitutes spiritual authority may prove to be a central dilemma for the Western student.

In the society out of which these sutras emerged, acceptance of the authority vested in tradition was a prerequisite for the serious spiritual aspirant. Most especially, that meant the authority of the Vedas. It also meant the authority of the spiritual teacher, who received his unquestioned authority from a lineage of vested predecessors. And within the long-standing socio-religious caste system in India, it meant the authority of the Brahmin priests as well.

In the West there has been a greater emphasis on empirical objectivity, with the result that science is frequently accorded greater authority than religion. In addition, the Western approach to spiritual teachings places a strong emphasis upon being relevant to contemporary experience and timely in terms of language. In this sense spiritual authority in the West is more equally shared between those who transmit teachings and those who receive them, as if prophet, priest, and layman enter into a mutually satisfactory understanding.

In determining who or what should be granted authoritative status, we in the West are likely to be concerned with the qualifications of the one claiming authority. So when a question of authority arises we tend to examine conditions which are external to us.

                    Sutra - 7

In Eastern culture, particularly in the spiritual realm, there is more emphasis placed upon one's receptiveness to authority, so when a question of authority arises there is a greater tendency to examine one's own internal conditions.

His Holiness the Dalai Lama once made the following suggestions in response to a seeker's question of how to choose a teacher or know a teacher to be reliable:

"This should be done in accordance with your interest and disposition, but you should analyze well. You must investigate before accepting a lama or guru to see whether that person is really qualified or not. It is said in a scripture of the Discipline (Vinaya) that just as fish that are hidden under the water can be seen through the movement of the ripples from above, so also a teacher's inner qualities can, over time, be seen a little through that person's behavior."

"We need to look into the person's scholarship – the ability to explain topics – and whether the person implements those teachings in his conduct and experience. [One teaching] says that you must investigate very carefully even if it takes twelve years. This is the way to choose a teacher." [15]

Chapter 1, Sutra 8
—— Offering ——

*Where you perceive from should not change
what you perceive,
unless you're in a dark room.*

- Jalal Al-din Rumi [16]

1.8 viparyayo mithyājñānamatadrūpapratiṣṭham

viparyayo mithyājñānamatadrūpapratiṣṭham

Translations

viparyaya - misperception; mistaking anything to
be reverse or opposite of what it is

from vi: - prefix meaning apart, in different
directions

+ paryaya: - 1. revolution (periodic)
2. contrariety, opposition
3. deviation from enjoined or
customary observances

mithya - conflicting, incorrect
(here: false)

(Continued)

---

jnana	-	knowledge
atadrupa (here: nonconformity)	-	not thus shaped, not so formed
pratishtam (here: based on)	-	1. standing still, resting, steadfastness 2. resting place, base, foundation

1.8 Misperception is false knowledge based on nonconformity (with its object).

—— Introductory Remarks ——

Misperception takes place when there is a lack of correspondence between a perceived object and the mind's sense-image of the object.

Since the misperceived object has real characteristics, there is always the possibility that sooner or later right knowledge will contradict false knowledge, and the object may then be correctly perceived. In the words of T.K.V. Desikachar:

> "Misapprehension is comprehension taken to be correct until more favorable conditions reveal the actual nature of the object. [It] is considered to be the most frequent activity of the mind." [17]

Misapprehension may occur through the operation of any of the other vrittis. That is, it may result from wrong perception or lack of perception, misunderstanding, a mistake in reasoning, a reliance on authority which is not reliable, illusory constructs of the mind, or mistaken memory.

viparyaya

One ancient commentator suggests that viparyaya arises "when there is what amounts to a memory, possessing a close similarity and conformity in time and place etc. to some thing." [18] The implication is that our preconceived notions or remembered experiences arising in an act of perception may adversely affect our capacity for accurate apprehension.

mithyajnanam

The root mith means to couple, encounter or engage in altercation. Mithya implies not just wrong or incorrect, but an incorrect coupling of two things. Mithyajnanam implies knowledge resulting from an incorrect coupling.

In the Kalki Purana, Mithya is personified as the wife of A-dharma (that which goes against one's highest duty.)

atadrupa

Atadrupa is translated here as nonconformity. It implies a comparison between two disparate things.

pratistham

Pratistham is a base, foundation or support. Here it refers to that upon which a mistaken cognition is based.

If we relate pratistham, which also means standing still or steadfast, to paryaya with its connotation of revolving, an image is suggested of remaining steadfast at one point in the mind's time and space continuum. In this context, this might suggest inappropriately holding onto one particular viewpoint or relationship to an object or event.

                    Sutra - 8

At any given moment we might have a viewpoint from which perception is based on a view that developed out of past experiences and does not correlate with present facts. Sometimes this viewpoint may be so strong and so persistent that it precludes correct apprehension.

Two Traditional Perspectives

"A man whose axe was missing suspected his neighbor's son. The boy walked like a thief, looked like a thief, and spoke like a thief. But the man found his axe while he was digging in the valley, and the next time he saw his neighbor's son, he walked, looked, and spoke like any other child."

- Traditional German Parable

"There is a kind of thought, which we call delusion... that leads [us] to become more fixed in the personality and fall further and further under the domination of the personality....A Sufi once said, 'We can't break natural law, but we can break our necks trying.' Is it possible that most of mankind is suffering from a maleficent delusion that causes us to be blind to the consequences of our actions?"

- Kabir Edmund Helminski, Living Presence [19]

———— Exploration ————

Inherent in the act of perception is point of view. Point of view is formed under the influence of many factors including location, conditions of the sense organs, emotional states, conceptual framework, memories and predispositions, motivations and intentions, and level of attention. Some of these formative factors may promote correct apprehension while others may inhibit it.

A point of view is complex, and because of this our comprehension of perceived objects is generally not just correct or incorrect, but a mixture: correct in one aspect and incorrect in another. Even when we are perceiving an object directly and under favorable conditions, this mixture is usually present.

When we are engaged in contemplation and most especially when we are contemplating subtleties such as meaning and significance, it is crucial to remember that our concepts are mixtures of many different ideas, some vague or faulty and some soundly based. We weave together these various threads, forming the fabric which clothes even our loftiest ideals. But in the process, we often lose sight of the individual threads.

We must also bear in mind the duality of relative truth and ultimate truth. From the perspective of relative truth, pramana may reveal some truth in regards to gross or subtle characteristics of the form nature, but still may fail to reveal the true essential nature of an object.

Ultimate truth, on the other hand, is not about personal perspective. Ultimate truth is true for every human being. The penultimate truth for us all is the unchanging nature of the pure awareness that exists behind the veils of the evolving personal self. In the course of an individual life, moments of ultimate truth are defined by the degree to which the obscuring veils of relative reality have been momentarily penetrated.

Our glimpses of ultimate truth set us firmly upon the spiritual path. We perceive some truth that transcends our normal daily lives and that truth acts as a magnet to pull us beyond the world of our personalities. But unless that transcendent truth becomes gradually integrated within our daily lives, transforming our personalities in the process, the majority of our experience will remain in relative awareness.

Integrating the relative with the ultimate is our task. It is a task that requires an ongoing purification and refinement of our relative experiential consciousness. When we cultivate our consciousness as we would a garden, with care and attention and hard work, with each season we see a more bountiful harvest. Patanjali is providing us with cultivation tools and setting out parameters so that we may begin to understand the workings of relative consciousness and better determine the course of our own growth.

—— Further Reflections ——

Within the context of the ancient spiritual traditions of India, the long-term maintenance and preservation of tradition far outweighs any consideration of keeping abreast of contemporary social concerns. In fact the preservation of tradition is so important that one of the conventional definitions of viparyaya is "deviation from enjoined or customary observances."

By contrast, in modern Western society, tradition often takes the back seat to social concerns of the times. It would probably be only a half-joke to suggest that a contemporary Western definition of viparyaya might be "blind adherence to enjoined or customary observances".

If we wish to come to a more universal understanding of the way viparyaya functions within the human mind, we must attempt to penetrate beneath the particular manifestations of social and cultural norms, ancient or contemporary.

In so doing, we perhaps may see that many of the problems inherent in the human mind are basically related to the fact that we have highly individuated minds that nonetheless operate within the context of a world mindstream. Any process we utilize in order to transform ourselves must take into account this basic dual nature of the mind.

We are in this way much like fish swimming in a stream: we are carried along by the stream's currents and are affected by its movements while also being affected by the other fishes. Yet the act of swimming can only be initiated through the life-force within each individual fish.

Ultimately every individual makes personal choices of belief and action based on their own perceptions of right and wrong. Even if the individual chooses to accept tradition or law as an absolute authority, this is nonetheless a personal decision based upon a perception of what is right and what is wrong. Even a refusal to engage in issues of right and wrong is a choice to move in one direction and avoid another direction. There is simply no way of avoiding the imperative of personal choice.

So we are faced with a situation where we must make choices, and these choices are necessarily dependent upon our point of view.

In yoga, point of view is of paramount concern, and ultimately the great challenge is to change the nature of our limited point of view. As part of that ongoing process, the challenge at any given moment is to not be unduly influenced by our personal point of view. This requires bearing in mind that not only do our perceptions include misperceptions, but also that we have limited means of immediately ascertaining their extent.

Fortunately, in the context of our spiritual practice, it is precisely this realization of the unreliable nature of the mind which leads us to find a deeper wisdom.

Chapter 1, Sutra 9
—— Offering ——

In the beginning was the word. Without thought,
invention, you would not have been, O Sword...
Without idea and the Word's mediation, you Would
have remained unmanifest in the dim dimension
where thought dwells...

- extract from The Walls Do Not Fall, by H.D. [20]

1.9 śabdajñānānupātī vastuśūnyo vikalpaḥ

śa̱bdajñā̱nā̱nupā̱tī vastuśūnyo̍ vika̱lpaḥ

Translations

sabda (here: word-sound)	-	1. sound, word, speech, language 2. verbal knowledge, verbal authority
jnana	-	knowledge, knowing
anupati	-	1. following upon, as a consequence of 2. proceeding in order
vastu	-	the real, any really existing or abiding substance, object, or essence

(Continued)

---

sunya	-	empty, void, absent
vikalpa	-	1. imagination, fancy
(here: imagination)		2. logic, thinking, conceptualization
		3. contrivance, art
		4. indecision, doubt, hesitation
from klrip:	-	to bear suitable relation, to correspond

1.9 Word (sound) and knowledge following upon absence of object is imagination.

—— Introductory Remarks ——

What is imagination?

The earliest sutra commentaries equated sabda and vikalpa with the transmission of "verbal testimony". While sabda differs from agama (scriptural authority), it was still sometimes classified as a pramana. Later analyses, however, present vikalpa as conceptualization or logical fallacies, not as valid means of pramana. Both approaches are valid in the context of Indian philosophy with its profound reliance on epistemological arguments.

But given the importance of creative imagination in contemporary culture, it would be remiss to limit this discussion to such a narrow framework.

Imagination is not only related to verbal testimony, conceptualizations or logical processes. It is the mechanism through which creativity and inspiration flows. It informs and shapes both the imaginative play of a child and the mature renderings of artist and musician, scientist and philosopher.

It is not only in our waking states that vikalpa occurs. Dreams are also imaginations. In fact, dreams are perhaps the most basic form of imagination, the process inherent in our physiological and psychological makeup that teaches us the process of how to create, how to bring inspiration into reality.

sabda

Sabda is a function of language, translated here as word (sound). It also refers to internalized words that have not been spoken aloud. An unuttered word or an unspoken thought can be even more powerful than their externalized counterparts.

Creativity is married to sabda as a means to focus intention within a given context. The creation stories of all religions revolve around sound as the basic means through which the creative force is initiated and directed.

jnana

Jnana means knowledge. In the context of vikalpa, jnana functions without external objective perception.

anupati

Anupati is translated as following upon.

vastu sunya

Vastu sunya may be translated as "without object" meaning that the object is not directly perceivable. The object may simply not be present. It may be non-objective such as God or purusa, or unmanifest (a child not yet conceived or a work of art not yet realized), a mythical entity (a mermaid or a unicorn), or an abstraction such as infinity.

vikalpa

Vikalpa is not as easy to define as the other four vrittis. The definition presented here is three-pronged:

vikalpa as   verbal testimony; conceptualizations; logical fallacies; doubt
vikalpa as   an image-making faculty; creativity
vikalpa as   dream

In our daily lives we regularly accept, at least on a temporary basis, an immense amount of verbal testimony and conceptualizations without proof of their correctness. Traditional examples of fallacies include assertions in which subject and predicate are by nature ill-suited to each other, such as "the attributes of purusa" (which has no attributes) or false attributes such as "the horn of a hare".

Another example of vikalpa may be described as a vague generalization. One modern commentator offers the phrase "the American way of life" as an example of this type of vikalpa.

Hariharananda Aranya's sutra commentary states: "There are expressions and words which have no answering reality. From hearing those words or expressions, an ideation takes place in our minds. This is a Vikalpa-vritti or modification due to vague notion. Those creatures who express their ideas through language have to depend largely on such notions. 'Ananta' (infinity) is an expression conveying a vague notion. We use that word often and understand its import to some extent. It is, however, not possible to comprehend the real significance of that word." [21]

In addition, there is the literal definition of vikalpa which merits consideration: vikalpa as doubt. Though not as common within yoga sutra commentaries, doubt is a widely accepted translation of vikalpa. Its usefulness is that it shows vikalpa as a mixed or fluctuating process of mind in which a given proposition viewed from one perspective appears to be correct, while from another perspective it appears to be incorrect.

—— **Exploration** ——

Imagination is the most complex of the five citta vritti and is the most difficult to penetrate, yet its comprehension is pivotal to an understanding of the human mind. Imagination lies at the very heart of the nature of the human mind. It is the wellspring of all the creativity, inventiveness and innovation of which we are capable as humans. It enables the vast array of mental constructs which we generate in response to thoughts and emotions. It enables the phenomenon of dreaming which is an integral part of our capacity to process and store what we learn. It allows us to use word symbols that become shorthand representations of the things we perceive. It encompasses ideation in its simplest form and extends to the most complex of concepts.

Without imagination, there would be no art, music, science, philosophy, psychology, mythology, religion.

It is worth noting that in yoga epistemology there are three basic elements involved in object perception:
artha (thing)
sabda (word)
jnana (knowledge)

In the act of direct perception, sense-images are generated in the mind as a more or less duplicative process. With sufficient comparison to their respective objects, these sense-images may then be determined to be correct or incorrect.

In vikalpa, since there is no "artha", the images of the mind are generated independent of any verifiable object, with language associations and concepts free to operate without the checks and balances of ordinary objective perception. In this way, the distinction between the real and the imaginary may be progressively blurred, leaving our minds increasingly under the guidance of our desires, wishes, feelings and emotions. Eventually, this may open the way for the rule of persuasion, charisma or greed.

In those avenues of thought where we are most likely to be passionate in our positions as, for example, in politics or religion, we are thus most vulnerable to being completely off-base.

Worse yet, since there is no short-term measure by which correct or incorrect may be judged, entire systems of thought or new social orders can be developed and put into practice without the realization that faulty basic premises have doomed them to failure from inception. Human history demonstrates all too well the devastating potential.

All this makes vikalpa a very fertile ground for development. Perhaps more than any other activity of the mind, by bringing attention to the vikalpa activities of the mind, we may begin the process of transformation of the citta vritti.

——— **Further Reflections** ———

To stimulate reflection on the relationship between artha, sabda, and jnana, we will briefly explore how the brain processes input of verbal and non-verbal data.

Names of objects as well as the ability to express verbal understanding of objects are language oriented tasks occurring primarily in the language sectors of the left side of the brain. The left side of the brain controls the right side of the body, and it is the strong predominance of the left-brain language sectors that accounts for the predominance of right-handedness amongst humans.

On the other hand, experiential knowledge for using or manipulating objects is generally handled within non-language sectors located within the right side of the brain, the side controlling the left side of the body.

When perception of an object occurs and the mind forms a sense-image of the object, that image usually includes two separate packets of data, language and non-language, handled respectively by the left and right sides of the brain. This verbal/non-verbal twosome also occurs when we imagine an object. So whether we see a cat or simply imagine a cat, two separate composite representations of cat, one verbal (left side) and one experiential (right side), are activated in the brain.

The verbal/non-verbal twosome is not, however, always bound together. Children, for example, accumulate a con-siderable bank of knowledge in regards to objects before they develop language skills; their learning process seems to proceed developmentally from perception to experiential representation, and then to language representation.

Even in adults, it is possible for verbal and non-verbal data to operate independently, as demonstrated clearly by medical cases involving single hemispheric brain damage. For example, an injured patient's verbal representations of an object may remain perfectly intact even after an injury to the brain has rendered the experiential counterpart no longer operative. In a case such as this, the patient may be able to identify and name an object such as a pen, or even converse coherently about it, without being able to access knowledge of what it is used for. [22]

This gives us some provocative food for thought. The interplay between the verbal and non-verbal images of the mind/brain complex is necessary within our normal manner of perceiving and communicating about objects. Consequently, a lack of balance between verbal and non-verbal brain functions may distort or obscure any object of our attention.

As a case in point, let us consider the traditional emphasis of yoga sutra commentaries in regards to vikalpa itself. Overwhelmingly, vikalpa is analyzed in relation to verbal processes. This likely reflects the general emphasis upon left hemisphere functions amongst highly educated persons.

But think for a moment about the implications. We have a word which is translated as imagination but is described and analyzed primarily in relation to words. Yet it is highly doubtful that any person, if asked to define their own personal experience of imagination, would define it as a word-centered activity.

Why the preoccupation with vikalpa and words? The left brain loves to talk and the right brain doesn't. Essentially, the left brain has a tendency to talk about itself and ignore the right brain (while the right brain silently observes) resulting in the nearly incessant chatter we tend to generate inside our heads. Anyone who has spent time listening to their own internal dialogue knows that vikalpa is one very active vritti, and one who has attempted to slow down the chatter more than momentarily knows the enormity of that task.

The fact remains, however, that the differences between left and right brain functions are more complex than a simple verbal/nonverbal dichotomy. Cognitive neuroscience provides us with some clues regarding the functioning of imagination within the human brain:

"It is believed that the two hemispheres of the human brain contribute to (conjured) imagery in rather different ways, the left hemisphere engaging essentially in an assembling of discriminated parts in order to construct a whole ('generative' mode), and the right hemisphere representing objects through a more wholistic mode, but without the subtle precision of detail of the left hemisphere. The 'generative' mode of the left hemisphere appears to be uniquely human, having evolved millions of years after the earlier wholistic mode of the right hemisphere." [23]

This model is especially interesting because of the close proximity, within the posterior left hemisphere, between the area implicated in 'generative' imagery and the areas responsible for language processing. There is ample evidence that adjacent processing centers within the brain are often functionally linked, and indeed there does appear to be a link between 'generative' image conjuring and language processing. This link might point to the route through which language is developmentally linked to the formation of imaginative and conceptual images. It might also account for the fact that the mind tends to busy itself with words even when it is engaged in direct perception. [24]

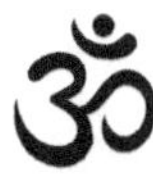

Chapter 1, Sutra 10
—— Offering ——

Good works lay upon my pillow
As upon an altar,
Mingling with heady blossoms of complacency
And the slow-burning incense "procrastinus".
My heart yearns for their release
But the Phoenix belongs to tomorrow.

- Margo Morris

1.10 abhāvapratyayālambanā tamovṛttirnidrā

abhāvapratyayālambanā tamovṛttirnidrā

<table>
<tr><td colspan="3"><h2 style="text-align:center">Translations</h2></td></tr>
<tr><td>abhava</td><td>-</td><td>non-existence, not-becoming, negation, absence</td></tr>
<tr><td>pratyaya
(here: seed-cognition)</td><td>-</td><td>1. ground, basis, motive, cause
2. cognition, idea</td></tr>
<tr><td>alambana</td><td>-</td><td>depending on, resting upon, having for its support</td></tr>
<tr><td>tamo</td><td>-</td><td>inertia, drowsy</td></tr>
<tr><td>(Continued)</td><td></td><td></td></tr>
</table>

vritti	-	processes (of the mind)
nidra	-	sleep, slumber, sloth

(here: dreamless sleep)

1.10 Dreamless sleep is the mental process which has for its support the seed-cognition of not becoming.

—— Introductory Remarks ——

Nidra refers to the mental activity of dreamless sleep in all its stages. In this state, outwardly directed conscious perception undergoes some form of suspension as the sense organs and the other vrittis are overcome by the vritti of sleep. Though dreaming is a state of consciousness that is normally entered only from a state of sleep, it is excluded here and classified instead as vikalpa.

abhava

Abhava is translated as not-becoming or absence. With regard to mental processes, abhava is the absence of the senses as well as the absence of the other four vrittis, which we identify as the experience of sleep.

pratyaya

Pratyaya has been translated variously as idea, notion, cognition, cause, or cognitive cause. The most misleading of these choices are idea and notion, implying as they do that a pratyaya is akin to a concept.

The translation used here is "seed-cognition", implying that a pratyaya is a core cognitive event that contains within itself the potential to bring forth more expanded cognitive events with similar content.

Perhaps the easiest way of beginning to understand the relation between vritti and pratyaya is to imagine an act of perception as a circuit that becomes established between the mind and its object.

As the mind moves outwards towards an object, it has a kind of intention-based "auto-select" search pattern which determines what types of data it will grasp and register. The basic core of this auto-select pattern, which helps determine the content of perception, is the pratyaya, the seed-cognition which arises within the mind as it reaches out to perceive. The mind then gathers to itself compatible information via one or more of the five vritti.

In this analogy the vrittis are like five giant digital search engines, while pratyaya is the search word. Information returned to the mind via the search engines interacts with pre-existing impressions and a succeeding pratyaya is generated to continue the outward circuit. When the pratyaya is highly focused, the entire circuit takes on that focus.

alambana

In the context of perception or meditation, alambana means "support". The support for the mind, when engaged in dreamless sleep, is abhava-pratyaya, the seed-cognition of not-becoming.

tamo

The word tamo is not usually included in this sutra, but in some traditions it is considered to be part of the text. It refers to the tamas guna of inertia.

     Sutra - 10

vritti

Of the five descriptions of the five vrittis, this is the only one that reiterates the term vritti. Perhaps it is not so readily obvious that sleep is a vritti and as such must be subject to nirodha along with the other vrittis. In addition, the reiteration of the term vritti serves to distinguish between sleep as a process of the mind and sleep as a physiological condition of the body.

nidra

Sleep is a periodic condition of the mind and body in which there is a suspension of external sensory perception and activities of the mind related to that perception, as well as suspension of the body's normal voluntary functions.

——— Exploration ———

By introducing the concept of pratyaya in this sutra, thus reminding us that the vritti of deep sleep is essentially no different from the other vrittis, Patanjali is bringing attention to the fact that the activities of the mind in normal sleep have the same core components as during the waking state.

At first glance it might appear that there is no "support" for the mind in deep sleep. To dispel this notion, Patanjali states that the normal activities of the mind in deep sleep are based upon abhava pratyaya (the seed-cognition of not-becoming).

Were this not the case, the nature of the mental experience of sleep would be quite different. If, for example, the pratyaya in deep sleep were nirodha, then sleep would be our defacto path to yogic transformation. And if there were no pratyaya in deep sleep, then sleep would constitute at least a temporary end to the misidentification of our true nature with the activities of the mind. Alas, our normal sense of self as well as our misidentification stays firmly intact as we slumber.

—— Further Reflections ——

Even though we generally spend about 30% of our lifetimes asleep, most of us are probably not very aware of what goes on during that time. Improving our awareness of our sleep and dream cycles is a good place to begin to come to terms with the fact that, as Patanjali has indicated, the mental activity of sleep is one of the five vrittis within our purview to transform.

During sleep both conscious awareness and sensory responsiveness are inhibited. Voluntary motor control is suspended and cerebral activity, respiration, heart rate and blood pressure are slowed. "Yet sleep is not a passive state: physiologically and neurologically, [it] is a complex state with distinct and predictable patterns, governed by an intrinsic rhythm of cyclic phases". [26]

The sleep cycle has two major components, REM (Rapid Eye Movement) sleep and non-REM sleep. Though REM sleep is classified here as vikalpa rather than nidra, it will serve us well to discuss the whole sleep cycle in one context.

"REM sleep is radically different than either deep sleep or the waking state. It is characterized subjectively by vivid dreaming, and objectively by muscle paralysis, with only the eye muscles remaining uninhibited. Non-REM sleep has four distinct cyclic stages. Entering the first stage of sleep from a waking state normally takes about 5-20 minutes. Each stage is characterized by a shift towards progressively lower frequency and higher amplitude brain waves, until after a total of about 50 minutes, the sleeper reaches the fourth stage of sleep, the stage technically referred to as deep sleep. During the descent from Stage 1 to Stage 4, muscle tone is still active and the sleeper will normally shift position several times."[27]

> "The next thing that happens...is that the stages reverse, progressing back from stage four to stage three [and so on]. Then one enters into a completely different state, the REM or paradoxical sleep that involves dreaming." In the first two to three hours of the night, "this pattern of passing through the four stages and back up again," and then into REM , persists. "The transition times are variable. What is not variable is that you cannot skip a stage...as dawn approaches, REM tends to predominate and deep sleep disappears."[28]

> "In REM sleep (the brain) is more active than in wakefulness....the upper brain, the forebrain, is very active electrically. In contrast to the waking state, this electrically active brain in the dreaming state is chemically distinct because of the shift in the neuro-transmitter ratios....we believe that this is very important for understanding the differences between the waking state and the dreaming state." [29]

Traditionally, the vritti of dreamless sleep is said to operate to the exclusion of the other vrittis. Current sleep research, however, points to the fact that there may be more activity of the mind in dreamless sleep than we normally recognize.

> "Even in going from awake to sleep, one sometimes has very brief flashes of imagery, called hypnagogic dreaming... when you wake people up from REM sleep, more than eighty percent say they were dreaming, and they can tell you what

they were dreaming about....It depends on how you evaluate the subjective report, but it is generally accepted that about half the people who are woken up from non-REM sleep report dreaming or mental activity. Many say they were thinking rather than dreaming. They report some kind of experience or mental activity, but it doesn't usually have the same full-fledged story quality as a dream....it is clearly true that vivid, visual storylike dreams occur classically in REM sleep." [30]

Transitions between waking and sleeping states are governed by the reciprocal aminergic and cholinergic systems in the brain stem which employ specific neurotransmitters (amino acids in the aminergic system, acetylcholine in the cholinergic) to control the succession of waking, sleeping and dreaming states.

"The cholinergic system is apparently held in restraint by the aminergic system. Thus, when the aminergic system is functioning at a high level, the cholinergic system is functioning at a reciprocally relatively low level. That is the situation in the waking state. As we go to sleep, the aminergic system decreases in its activity, and the cholinergic system becomes progressively more active throughout the periods of deep sleep without dream...the cholinergic system reaches its highest level of activity just when you enter the dream state ....activation of the cholinergic cells generates signals that contribute to eye movements, to inhibition of muscle tone, and activation of the forebrain", all indicators of the REM state." [31]

There may be a great deal we can learn about meditative states by studying states of sleep. For example, the aminergic and cholinergic systems which control our waking and sleeping cycles also exert control over our levels of alertness, arousal, and anxiety in the waking state. These systems also regulate our flow of energy and affect such vital functions as respiration and blood pressure. It has even been suggested that the proper regulation of

the aminergic system is one of the goals of meditative practices.
[32]

If this is indeed the case, a strong possibility exists that many of the advanced meditative practices which have been passed down to us through tradition will be better understood as we develop the technology which will allow for objective observation.

In the meantime, much can be gained by simply observing our states of consciousness as we fall asleep, in the same way that we observe as we meditate. One simple observation that is easy to witness is that in falling asleep the mind continues to register images in much the same way as when entering into meditation. The major difference is that in meditation these images are usually tempered by an intentional control or restraint.

Sutra - 10

Chapter 1, Sutra 11
—— Offering ——

By some mystery, the tree of childhood wonder
Took root within my mind.
Half a century of spring blossoms
Have risen from this fertile soil.
How odd, it never thought to bear a single peach.

- Margo Morris

1.11 anubhūtaviṣayāsaṃpramoṣaḥ smṛtiḥ

anubhūtaviṣayāsaṃpramoṣaḥ smṛtiḥ

Translations

anubhuta	-	perceived, experienced
from anubhu:	-	to enclose, to perceive, understand, experience
visaya	-	1. sphere (of influence); scope, range 2. an object of sense; impression
asampramosa	-	not stealing away
from mush:	-	1. to steal, carry off, deprive of 2. to cloud, obscure

(Continued)

---

smrti	-	1. memory
		2. that which is remembered
		3. traditional sacred texts

1.11 Memory is the not stealing away of experienced objects.

—— Introductory Remarks ——

Memory is the retention and recall of images formed under the influence of the other vrittis.

anubhuta

What has been perceived or embraced by the mind is anubhuta.

visaya

Visaya indicates specific objects of experience as well as the sphere of experience as a whole.

asampramosa

This is a curious and enigmatic choice of terms. The translation is generally given as "not stealing away". What exactly is not stolen away? Vyasa posed the question: "Does the mind remember the act of knowing or the object?"

In this study we are working from the premise that the act of knowing always involves the formation of a mental image which is distinct from the object perceived. This mental image is formed with the aid of the senses but, being influenced by the totality of the individual's point of view, is something much more than just the impressions received by the brain directly from the eyes, ears, etc.

In considering the meaning of asampramosa we must consider the reliability of sources and examine what constitutes authenticity of experience. For if we cannot distinguish between memories of our experience, memories of our imaginings, and memories of what we have gleaned from the experience of others, we will not be well-positioned to refine and purify the contents of our memory storehouse.

smrti

Memory is a process in which images formed by the mind under the influence of the other vrittis are retained and then accessed again at a later time. Recalled images may not be faithful to the original experience. It is usually the case that the vivid precision of detail and the capacity for scrutiny which are the hallmarks of direct perception, are not available to the same extent in memory.

Within the spiritual traditions of the East, there is also a broader meaning of smriti wherein it refers to the entire body of authoritative spiritual texts passed down from generation to generation.

Two views of Memory

Memory is astonishing and elusive -- its threads intricately woven and infinitely complicated. It makes intelligible the chaos of experience; it feeds our creativity and shapes our daily judgments, our spiritual apprehensions, our desires. It is the essential element of human consciousness, the key to our personality, and the linchpin of our sense of who we are...memory unifies disparate experiences, creates a synthesis...and binds together a self, a family, a culture, and indeed all humanity. [33]

- James McConkey, The Anatomy of Memory

"Were you ever instructed by a wise and eloquent man? Remember then, were not the words that made your blood run to your cheeks, that made you tremble or delighted you, -- did they not sound to you as old as yourself?... It is God in you that responds to God without, or affirms his own words trembling on the lips of another. [34]

- Ralph Waldo Emerson

$$\text{------ } \textbf{Exploration} \text{ ------}$$

Historically, both the study and practice of yoga has placed great emphasis upon the training of memory. Until recent times, memory was the primary tool for the transmission of the teachings of yoga from generation to generation. This undoubtedly stemmed at least in part from a deep understanding of the fact that in order to transform the activities of the mind, it is necessary to influence the way in which memory functions.

Memory is the river upon which self-awareness flows. Our self-image and personal history are boats upon that river. Without memory, there could be no sense of continuity in consciousness, there could be no learning. Memory links our self-awareness to our experiential context of past, present and future.

If we contemplate the nearly inexpressible complexity of our own self-image and the ever-malleable conglomeration of impressions that we string together to form our own personal history, we may gain some insight into the nature of the vritti called memory.

"...Memory not only re-creates the past, but must be the source of the future as well, because all our salients into the future are built upon what we know from the past, and what we fancy from it. Conferring with memory's ghosts, consulting its tables of facts, we project the future and what we expect it to look like. Memory makes us, fore and aft." [35]

Once mental images have been formed in relation to a particular object, those images are reactivated by the mind whenever new images bear a sufficient resemblance. In addition, subjective experience tells us that the act of remembering is usually accompanied by an awareness of the present moment in which remembering occurs. This suggests that even during an act of remembering, new memories are being formed even as old ones are accessed.

How does this intermingling of past and present affect us as yoga practitioners?

The natural interplay between our memories and our current perceptions offers an always present opportunity for comparison and reevaluation. If used well, this can be developed into a "moment of reflection" which has a profound potential as a tool for growth.

—— Further Explorations ——

Memory as an act of data retrieval is unpredictable. When information is stored in memory it is not possible to know for certain whether or not that particular data will be capable of being recalled at a later date or how accurate the recall will be. Furthermore, one successful retrieval is not necessarily an indication that the next attempt will be equally successful.

"It has been shown just how delicate memory is, how fickle and changeable, as it forms and reforms after the fact. It has become clear that the act of memory is an act of construction, not of recording. That is, we create memory as we go, rather than being mere registers of the events around us. We reshape memory as we move through experience, and reshape experience with expectations brought up from memory...Our perceptions, memories, and the thoughts which arise out of their interaction are reflected and re-reflected among our mental mirrors." [36]

Just like every other vritti, memory has its roots within the physical brain. Memory functions by carving actual pathways in the physical terrain of the brain. Traffic-wise, certain roads within the memory terrain of the brain are well traveled. Others are less traveled. Experience tells us that the memory paths we most commonly travel do not necessarily lead to places we would consciously choose to visit if we really took the time to consider.

"The brain is constantly remodeling its own physical structure to reflect how it is being used. Moment by moment we choose how we will behave in the present and the future, and these choices are embossed on the physical material of our minds." [37]

Our potential for reorganizing and reinterpreting the perceptual, conceptual and experiential data of our own minds is a real one. In our work to transform the vrittis, we should recognize just how important the transformation of memory is, and how crucial it is in the interplay between our relative and ultimate perspectives on reality.

The interplay between memory and current perception, utilized properly, gives us a chance not only to reevaluate our perspective, but to identify and consciously change the most basic underlying patterns of functioning within our minds.

Chapter 1, Sutra 12
—— *Offering* ——

My attention is a wild animal;
It will if idle make trouble
where there was no harm...

- A. R. Ammons, extract from "Pet Panther" [38]

1.12 abhyāsavairāgyābhyaṁ tannirodhaḥ

abhyāsavairāgyābhyāṃ tannirodhaḥ

Translations

abhyasa — repeated exercise or discipline
(here: practice)

from abhyas: — 1. to throw towards or upon
2. to concentrate attention upon

vairagya — (case ending: abhyam -Inst. dual)
1. dispassion, non-attachment
2. detachment

from vai: — 1. to become weary or exhausted
2. to be deprived of

+ raga: — passion or vehement desire

(Continued)

---

tan	-	that, this
(here: these)		
nirodha	-	1. restraint, confinement, enclosure
(here: harnessing)		2. sprouting, growing, sowing, ascending

1.12 Harnessing of these
through practice and dispassion.

—— Introductory Remarks ——

After enumerating and describing the five normal processes of the mind, we now turn to a discussion of how nirodha may be achieved through practice and dispassion, in what may be described as a process of subtilization and transformation.

abhyasa

Abhyasa means repetition. In this context, it refers to the repeated and continual use of any practice or discipline through which some degree of control over the normal processes of the mind is established.

vairagya

It is not easy to communicate an accurate sense of the meaning of vairagya. It is translated here as dispassion, though the desired meaning is more like fervent equanimity than an absence of passion. Yet we are accustomed to equating passion with desire for worldly pleasures and in this sense the term dispassion serves well.

Another way of looking at vairagya is in relation to the klista/

aklista description of the vrittis (sutra 1.5). When we say that a certain vritti is klista or aklista, what we are measuring is our own personal emotional response in relation to that process.

Klista/aklista is the symptom; vairagya is the antidote. One modern writer on the sutras, Bernard Bouanchaud, comments:

[Vairagya] "implies a certain kind of freedom from emotions and sentiment. (It) signifies the stability and serenity that arise when we withdraw from passion... the less we identify with our passions, the greater is our inner peace in spite of difficulties." [39]

Vijnana Bhiksu states:

"Dispassion is not mere negation of passion or attachment; for in that case the epithet "dispassioned" would apply to one who has no passion for an object away from him (and as such not inviting his attention)." [40]

abhyam

For the most part, grammatical issues such as case endings are not being addressed in this study. In this instance, however, the implication of the case ending abhyam is particularly relevant. Abhyam is a dual case ending that is used in denoting an integrated pair, thus indicating that neither practice nor dispassion alone are sufficient to the task; both are necessary for the cultivation of nirodha.

tan

Tan (these) refers here to the normal processes of the mind, as enumerated and explained in the previous seven sutras.

nirodha

Yoga is defined as citta vritti nirodha. The five types of citta vritti may all be experienced as klista or aklista. Practice and dispassion are the means of nirodha.

Here nirodha is defined as harnessing. As we proceed, it may also be useful to think of nirodha in terms of the processes of subtilization and transformation -- subtilization through practice and transformation through dispassion.

—— Exploration ——

In our context, practice is the intentional repetition of some set of prescribed actions, either gross or subtle, in order to influence the citta vritti. As such, practice is the means by which we direct and reinforce our commitment to our spiritual growth.

Dispassion is a diminishing susceptibility to the various emotions and attractions which perpetuate the normal habitual activities of the mind. Dispassion is a result of our desire to loosen the bonds of our emotional and worldly entrapments, making available to us the power to discern what is actually conducive to our growth.

Any kind of deep and lasting change requires a fresh perspective and new ways of behaving, It also requires the ability to discern and abandon that which is no longer useful. These requirements can be related to practice, which includes aspects of conscious choice, commitment, discipline, and action. There is a certain linear quality to practice; functionally, it is a more or less ordered and step-by-step process. The subtilization aspect of nirodha is strongly linked to successful practice.

Dispassion, by comparison, is a less linear process. Dealing as it does with the fluidity of our feeling/desire nature, it demonstrates more as a result than as an immediately accessible choice. It is the fertile field in which the process of transformation takes place. Vairagya may show itself in small and ordinary ways, or in ways that are quite extraordinary.

In thinking about practice and dispassion, and in attempting to understand both the distinctions between them and the manner in which they are intertwined, it is useful to consider the nature of attention. What is capable of capturing our attention? What is worthy of attention? How can we direct our attention and sustain it in a particular direction, and how does this process affect the quality of available attention?

Since we are often "led by the nose" of our desires and sense attractions, what gets our attention is not necessarily what we would consciously claim to be most worthy. Expediency may also guide our attention, and therefore our actions, against our better judgment. Likewise, the path of least resistance lays its claim, though habit may well be a stronger pull simply because of its familiar terrain. The prime mover of attention, however, is probably avoidance of discomfort and pain.

When we have a conscious desire for change and are ready to make some kind of change, what we often have to deal with first is whatever is causing us immediate suffering, even if it seems rather trivial. For whatever they may be, our immediate sufferings offer us a place to start that is real within the context of our current experience, thus lending a certain solidity to our work.

Starting small may be a good strategy. For example, if we begin our process of change by placing our attention on simple and obvious sufferings such as a shoulder pain, we may be able to temporarily bypass some of the conceptual confusions that often surround more "meaningful" issues. In this way, we may be able to quickly learn certain principles related to attention and transformation, and actually make more headway than if we were to move directly towards bigger challenges without the necessary preparation.

The idea in developing a practice is to bring our intelligent awareness to some present condition we want to change. We start by observing how our habit patterns reinforce the condition. Then we introduce some conscious action that disrupts the normal course of our actions and attitudes. This procedure shifts our perspective if only in a small way. It is this shift of perspective that is the raison de etre of practice, for once our perspective changes, our condition very simply is no longer the same.

Why then is practice alone not enough? If we can actually effect changes in our condition and develop a fresh perspective through our practice, why then is dispassion a necessary ingredient?

The answer lies in the very nature of our learning process as humans. We possess an incredible potential for learning, but our capacity for destructive behavior patterns equals our capacity for constructive ones. Because of this, even while in the midst of establishing practices geared towards positive change, we will inevitably be pulled in directions that are, shall we say, less positive, being grounded in desires that serve to maintain the status-quo of our self-centeredness. Vyasa states in his commentary: "The river of the mind-field indeed flows both ways. It flows towards beatitude and it flows towards evil." [41]

Dispassion enables us to stem the tide of the habitual desires and habitual attitudes and behaviors in which we no longer wish to engage. Without dispassion, the possibility exists that as we gain strength and stability in our practice, our newfound strength will actually lend its power to the aspects of our personality which are primarily self-serving. We may, in this way, reinforce destructive habits and limit our potential for developing a more inclusive perspective. We may also unwittingly develop obsessions in regard to our practice.

These are concerns to be taken quite seriously. It is likely that many of us know at least one person who has, through spiritual practice, actually strengthened his or her arrogance, conceit, or need to dominate others. When this occurs, the perverted personal power of the unfortunate practitioner is sometimes so cleverly disguised and so well-defended that a great deal of destruction may come to pass before the path is set straight.

—— Further Reflections ——

Whenever we want to head in a new direction, we need a healthy measure of self-reflection in order to assess our situation clearly. When we are consciously creating new parameters for ourselves and cultivating new modes of behavior, it is wise to maintain some measure of order and stability in order to assure a successful transition.

It may be useful to look at the interdependence of practice and dispassion through the lens of the dual hemisphere nature of the human brain with its system of checks and balances.

In the dual-hemisphere system there is a great deal of lateral specialization. Much of what science has been able to glean about this specialization has come to light through the study of localized pathologies and injuries of the brain.

One such study concerns a medical condition termed anosognosia, literally "unaware of illness". This condition is observed in a small minority of patients who have some paralysis on the left side of the body after a stroke that has damaged the right hemisphere. A patient with anosognosia will typically ignore or even completely deny the fact of their own paralysis. Even when challenged to move a paralyzed arm or leg these patients will stay in denial, offering reasons as to why they are unable to move the limb at present, and often maintaining rationalizations to a point of absurdity. [42]

The most obvious explanation of anosognosia is that the patient is simply unable to accept the reality of the trauma which has occurred. But this psychological explanation does not address the fact that this type of denial syndrome is almost always associated with damage to only one side of the brain - the right hemisphere - resulting in paralysis of the body's left side. When people suffer damage to the left hemisphere, resulting in paralysis on the body's right side, this type of denial rarely occurs. [43]

Dr. V.S. Ramachandran, a neuroscientist who has worked extensively in the research and treatment of unusual neurological conditions, offers a theory for the anosognosia denial syndrome that delves deeply into the mysteries of bilateral specialization within the brain, and in so doing shines a light on the psychological functioning of each and every one of us. Elaborating on the fact that the left hemisphere is specialized for language while the right hemisphere is concerned with more holistic aspects of communication, including the ability to respond with appropriate emotion to evocative situations, Dr Ramachandran writes:

"In addition to these obvious divisions of labor, I want to suggest an even more fundamental difference between the cognitive styles of the two hemispheres, one that not only helps explain the amplified defense mechanism of anosognosia but may also help account for the more mundane forms of denial that people use in daily life - such as when an alcoholic refuses to acknowledge his drinking problem or when you deny your forbidden attraction to a married colleague."

"At any given moment in our waking lives, our brains are flooded with a bewildering array of sensory inputs, all of which must be incorporated into a coherent perspective that's based on what stored memories already tell us is true about ourselves and the world. In order to generate coherent actions, the brain must have some way of sifting through this superabundance of detail and of ordering it into a stable and internally consistent "belief system" – a story that makes sense of the available evidence. Each time a new item of information comes in we fold it seamlessly into our preexisting worldview. I suggest that this is mainly done by the left hemisphere."

"[If] something comes along that does not quite fit the plot, what your left hemisphere does...is either ignore the anomaly completely or distort it to squeeze it into your preexisting framework, to preserve stability...."

"The right hemisphere's strategy, on the other hand, is to play "Devil's Advocate", to question the status quo and look for global inconsistencies. When the anomalous information reaches a certain threshold, the right hemisphere decides that it is time to force a complete revision of the entire model and start from scratch. The right hemisphere thus forces a "Kuhnian paradigm shift" in response to anomalies, whereas the left hemisphere always tries to cling tenaciously to the way things were." [44]

To test his theory, Dr. Ramachandran performed many ingenious experiments with patients who suffer from anosognosia. One experiment devised by an Italian neurologist involved irrigating the denial patient's left ear canal with cold water, setting up a convection current in the ear canals and thus causing involuntary correctional eye movements which somehow reorient the brain.

The results of this experiment are nothing less than astonishing. If, after the procedure, the patient is questioned about his paralyzed limb, the patient will readily admit to the paralysis. But the admittance is only short term. Within a period of hours the patient will not only resume his denial, but will apparently have no memory of having previously admitted to being paralyzed. [45]

Now, what does all this have to do with abhyasa and vairagya?

First of all, it points towards the possibility of a deeper understanding of the neurological underpinnings of our cognitive and emotional states.

In addition, investigations such as this provide us with a novel way of looking at our own internal coping strategies. One of the advantages of understanding our own psychic mechanisms at a level of brain functions, is that it tends to neutralize the very human tendency to react with defensiveness or guilt or shame when faced with our own personal rationalizations and denials.

If, within our own processes of self-discovery, we can begin to view the dual propensities of our human nature as being hard-wired, so to speak, and yet still hold the vision of the profound evolutionary potentials of our human nature, perhaps we may find it a bit easier to muster the courage and persistence we need for our spiritual growth.

Chapter 1, Sutra 13
—— *Offering* ——

Find a way to your innermost secret.
Let no other perception distract you.
You, yourself, possess the elixir,
so rub it into your skin, and by this alchemy
your inner enemies will become friends.

- Jalal Al-din Rumi. extract from "Open the Window" [46]

1.13 tatra sthitau yatno 'bhyāsaḥ

tatra sthitau yatno'bhyāsaḥ

Translations

tatra	-	1. therein, in that 2. of these
sthitau	-	1. standing, staying, resting, abiding 2. steadiness, stability
yatno (here: willful effort)	-	1. activity of will, volition 2. effort, exertion, work
abhyasa	-	practice (see 1.12)

1.13 Practice is the willful effort towards steadiness in that (nirodha).

—— Introductory Remarks ——

As defined here, practice (abhyasa) is a volitional effort towards steadiness of control over the normal processes of the mind.

tatra

Tatra references the previous sutra. It has been interpreted in various ways, including "between these" (abhyasa and vairagya) and "in this" (nirodha).

sthitau

Sthitau is a form of the word sthiti, meaning stability.

A certain steadiness or calm, undisturbed flow of the mind (thoughts, emotions, feelings, energy) is perhaps the first observable manifestation that some degree of control of the normal processes of the mind has been achieved. With increased control comes increased steadiness.

yatno

Yatno means effort or exertion, but it also means volition or will, thus the translation as "willful effort".

Practice involves conscious choice and commitment, actions which support this commitment, and an ongoing effort towards mindfulness.

abhyasa

To be effective, the effort expended in practice as well as the particulars of practice must be well suited to the individual practitioner. Even then, steadiness is not easily achieved.

Swami Veda Bharati in his commentary states:

"It is a common experience that whatever depth of meditation one reaches remains a temporary experience at first. No sooner does one reach it during a meditation session than he or she slips down, and during the activity of daily life meditative depth remains elusive. Only by continuous application of will and constancy of practice does it become possible for one to learn to "remain there" at first during the meditation, and later to maintain that depth in daily life." [47]

A Perspective From Buddhist Tradition

"Although my experience may be very little, one thing that I can say for certain is that I feel that through Buddhist training, I feel that my mind has become much more calm. That's definite. Although the change has come about gradually, perhaps centimeter by centimeter, I think that there has been a change in my attitude towards myself and others."

"Although it's difficult to point to the precise causes of this change, I think that it has been influenced by a realization, not full realization, but a certain feeling or sense of the underlying fundamental nature of reality, and also through contemplating subjects such as impermanence, our suffering nature, and the value of compassion and altruism." [48]

- H.H. The Dalai Lama

——— Exploration ———

What constitutes practice?

In the West, the practice of yoga has by and large been equated with the practice of asana, the physical postures of yoga. The configurations of the body in asana range from simple to complex. The most basic approach to asana is a structural, bio-mechanical approach utilizing postures to correct misalignments and imbalances.

Asana practice is also a powerful tool for maintaining the physiological systems of the body as well as integrating and reorganizing the subtle energy systems. Within a well designed asana practice we have the opportunity to bring our conscious awareness to a more unified experience of our mental, emotional, energetic and physical "bodies", which we normally experience as more compartmentalized than they actually are.

An asana practice may also serve as a springboard to more subtle elements of practice. Ideally, the student of asana learns that there are principles and methodologies that can be utilized to produce transformation, and then goes on to apply analogous principles and methodologies with the use of more subtle components of yoga such as pranayama, chanting and mantra, contemplation, and meditation.

In a focused practice, the chosen object of attention may be the spine, the breath, a mantra, some intuitive insight, compassion, or a higher power. The quality of attention is not necessarily demonstrated by the choice of object, though generally the more subtle objects require more refined attention.

Practice is seen to be the application of principles and methodology, and the chosen methodology should address the needs of the individual.

Regardless of the specifics of an individual's practice, however, there is one primary goal which rightfully becomes its guiding force. That goal is to bring the full attention of the mind to the practice. The ultimate intention of practice is to harness attention, and when this intention is clear and strong, one gains the ability to concentrate one's mind effectively.

—— Further Reflections ——

One of the natural outcomes of a regular yoga practice is some degree of reorientation in what we consider to be klista and aklista.

This reorientation comes about through a combination of intention, action, and a shift of perspective which includes a shift in our way of looking at ourselves. This process might be described as follows:

1. we desire to change
2. we come to an understanding that change is possible
3. we make a commitment to change
4. finally, we put change into practice

What happens in yoga practice is no different from what happens when we make any kind of change, even a simple one such as a change in diet. When we adopt a new diet we may at first have some resistance or frustration. We may even be tempted to abandon our new discipline and indulge in a craving even if it is hazardous to our health. But if we persist with the new diet, what we inevitably find is that our tastes simply change. What we like and what we don't like somehow get redefined. For some of us, looking back at our eating habits of five, ten, or fifteen years ago, it may be hard to believe that we ever actually wanted to eat the way we did. Yet we did want to. And now we don't.

In the same way, as we persist in our yoga practice, we may notice changes in our lifestyle. We may develop new perspectives on how we want to care for our bodies and how we want to conduct our relationships. We may notice, quite literally, changes in the way we think and feel.

If we are diligent, we might become more aware of the repetitive rhythms of the mindstream as it loops its way through the landscape of our consciousness, alternately forming rapids and reservoirs.

We might observe that the emotional content of the mindstream is not so much spontaneous as it is predictably inconsistent. Most probably we will also observe that for all the inconsistency of the emotional content, the verbal content of the mindstream is astonishingly repetitive.

As we come to realize that the activities of our minds are both repetitive and inconsistent, chances are we will begin to welcome opportunities to step off the merry-go-round long enough to regain a sense of balance. Through our practice we consciously cultivate these opportunities.

Once established, practice carves out a path for itself, ever deepening and ever widening, as we come to cherish the calmness and tranquility of its flow.

Sutra - 13

Chapter 1, Sutra 14
—— *Offering* ——

O precious Flame lighting my heart,
Waxing and waning evermore in
Rhythmical two-step with
The shadow dancers in my mind.
Faithfully following, step by step,
This cosmic dance.
How I long for you to take the lead.

- Margo Morris

1.14 sa tu dīrghakālanairantaryasatkārādarāsevito
dṛḍhabhūmiḥ

sa tu dīrghakālanairantaryasatkārādarāsevito dṛḍhabhūmiḥ

Translations		
sa	-	this
tu	-	but, then, however, now
dirgha	-	long, for a long time
kala	-	time
nairantarya	-	uninterrupted, continuous
(Continued)		

satkara	-	reverence, honor, devotion
adara	-	respect, care, attentiveness
asevito	-	1. frequented, visited often 2. performed assiduously
drdha	-	1. firm, steady, resolute 2. established, certain 3. anything fixed or firm (a stronghold, fortress)
bhumi	-	1. earth, ground 2. step or stage (within a process)

1.14 Now this (practice) is on firm ground when performed assiduously, with attentiveness and devotion for a long time, uninterruptedly.

—— Introductory Remarks ——

This sutra offers some practical guidelines for a successful practice. The indication is that consistency and regularity, as well as the quality of intention and attention which one brings to one's practice, are the determining factors for establishing that practice on a solid footing.

sa tu

Sa tu refers to abhyasa, or practice.

dirgha kala

Kala refers to time as a general phenomenon but also expresses specific, fixed points in time, and in addition may carry the connotation of appropriate points in time. Dirgha means 'long' in time or space. The simplest rendering of dirgha kala is 'long time'.

nairantarya

Dirgha kala nairantarya translates as "for a long time uninterruptedly" or "regularly, without fail".

satkara

Kara is from the verbal root "kr" meaning to do or to make. "Sat" in this context carries the meaning of right, proper, as it ought to be. Traditionally satkara expresses a quality of devotion, reverence, honor and humility in following prescribed religious observances.

adara

The word adara, though it does not appear in many yoga sutra texts, is considered within some traditions to be a part of the text. Adara implies respect, especially in the form of careful attentiveness to detail.

asevito

Asevito is derived from a root which means to frequent or abide in. Taken in context with dirgha kala nairantarya, it may point towards discreet (perhaps fixed) periods of regular practice. Alternatively it could be taken to suggest practice of a more continuous nature, with a more or less uninterrupted flow over an extended period of time, as in "practicing the presence of God."

drdha bhumi

Drdha bhumi means on firm ground or in steady steps.

Through one of the shades of meaning of drdha (see above translations), the image of a fortress, which we encountered in sutra 1.2 in connection with nirodha, is once again invoked.

A Christian Perspective

"Our wills are ours and it is our wills that affect all that we do by willing, and which would not have happened if we had not willed...but the power of achievement comes from God."

- Saint Augustine, The City Of God [49]

—— Exploration ——

The elements of a practice should be determined after careful consideration of one's actual needs. Equally important to the success of a practice is the attitude and attentiveness with which it is approached. Even a well designed practice cannot bear the full fruit of its potential without the cultivation of inner states that are conducive to transformation.

The ability to direct and maintain one's attention to the particular requirements of a practice is not a simple task. It requires enthusiasm, self-confidence, commitment, and an understanding that growth takes place gradually over time through continual effort and refinement.

An inner attitude of humility and reverence (satkara) must also be cultivated. Satkara is the fountainhead of wisdom and inspiration which empowers us to diminish our identification with the activities of the mind and eventually develop the ability to control those activities as desired. Through humility and reverence we are able to loosen the bonds of our ego attachments and strengthen our connectedness to our own highest vision of truth.

As Swami Rama has reminded us:

"Selflessness is one common characteristic that we find among all great men and women of the world. Nothing could be achieved without selfless service. All the rituals and knowledge of the scriptures are in vain if actions are performed without selflessness." [50]

As for persistence and regularity, they are necessary requirements of any learned discipline. One must have the fortitude to overcome periods of frustration and self-doubt, as well as their flip-side, cockiness and pride.

—— Further Reflections ——

Practice is a discipline encompassing many different methodologies which may be applied to a wide range of intended goals. In the present context we should bear in mind that Patanjali is speaking of practice as a means of controlling the vrittis. For it is the "harnessing" of the vrittis which is defined as yoga.

The harnessing of the vrittis need not, however, be the immediate focus of a practice. The activities of the mind may be affected directly or indirectly, and it is important to remember that no mater what kind of practice we do, every level of our being is affected.

For example, we might be attempting to work out a structural or physiological problem through asana, or to redirect our emotional energy through ritual and contemplation, or to coordinate the subtle energies of the body through breath practices. Such particular focuses are powerful in determining the effects of a practice, but we are integrated beings and what we do affects our entirety.

In fact, one of the means of assessing effectiveness in practice is to carefully observe all effects, as equilibrium should ideally be enhanced at every level. Practice at its best promotes well-being for the whole person.

Having taken this into account, the fact remains that if control of the vrittis is to be a significant part of our goal we must practice such control assiduously, recognizing that both the cognitive aspects and emotional aspects of the vrittis must be regulated. Our thoughts, our feelings, and every aspect of our relationship to our perceptions must be brought within the arena of our conscious influence.

When we choose to exercise control of the activities of our own minds, we are choosing nothing less than transformation of the very nature of our personhood, and must be prepared to persevere despite the multitude of obstacles that will inevitably arise.

Chapter 1, Sutra 15
—— *Offering* ——

Of all that God has shown me
I can speak only the smallest word,
Not more than a honey bee
Takes on his foot from an overspilling jar.

- Mechtild of Magdeburg [51]

1.15 dṛṣṭānuśravikaviṣayavitṛṣṇasya
vaśīkārasaṁjñāvairāgyam

dṛṣṭānuśravikaviṣayavitṛṣṇasya vaśīkārasaṁjñāvairāgyam

Translations

drsta	-	seen, that which is perceptible
anusravika	-	heard about, that which is known through tradition
from anu:	-	prefix meaning after, according to
+ sravika:	-	hearing, learning
visaya	-	1. sphere (of influence); scope 2. an object of sense; impression

(Continued)

vitrsnasya	-	one who is free from desire
vasikara (here: self-mastery)	-	lit. "willing-doing" subjugating, subject to will
samjna (here: quality of clear consciousness)	-	1. consciousness, clear knowledge 2. agreement, mutual understanding
vairagyam	-	dispassion (see 1.12)

1.15 Dispassion is the quality of clear consciousness (arising from) the self-mastery of one who is free from desire for objects seen or heard about.

—— Introductory Remarks ——

Having clarified the meaning of practice (abhyasa) in the previous two sutras, Patanjali now presents two sutras on the subject of dispassion (vairagya).

Dispassion is defined as a certain quality of consciousness achieved through self-mastery, exhibiting as a freedom from thirst for any object, gross or subtle.

drsta

Drsta means seen, and refers to gross objects perceptible through the five senses, but also carries the connotation of worldly objects as opposed to sacred objects.

anusravika

Anusravika literally means "after hearing" or "after learning".

Here the term refers to objects of a subtle nature, especially experiences or accomplishments such as siddhis (powers) or "heavenly" experiences such as those described in sacred teachings.

visaya

Visaya indicates specific objects as well as the sphere of experience as a whole.

vitrsnasya

A vitrsnasya is one who is free from craving. Vitrsna, free of thirst, is often translated as indifference. This can carry the implication of dullness or aloofness, which runs counter to the intended meaning.

We must also consider that freedom from craving may arise from various causes. For example, a sick person will naturally exhibit a temporary loss of certain cravings; prior to puberty one may be relatively indifferent to the opposite sex; a young person may not have yet developed greed or a craving for power. But these are not indications that a freedom from craving has been achieved.

The implication here is that one acquires a freedom from craving through personal experiences which lead to the ability to discern what is conducive to growth and what is not conducive to growth.

Swami Hariharananda states:

"The difference between getting to know about the demerit of things through study and reflection alone and the wisdom through discriminative knowledge is like the difference in experience between hearing that fire burns and actually getting burnt." [52]

vasikara

Vasikara is a compound term from two roots: vas (to will) and kr (to do). It literally means "willing-doing", implying an interaction between will and action. This provides us with a hint as to methodology. It is through what might be called "willful acquiescence" that self-mastery is achieved.

samjna

Samjna means consciousness or clear knowledge, and is applied to a person who has a particular level of clarity. Samjna combined with vasikara frequently renders a translation of "consciousness of mastery", though the meaning of such a translation is ambiguous. For example, consciousness of ethics is not at all the same as ethical consciousness. By reversing the traditional order of the two translated terms, rendering "mastery of consciousness", the intended meaning is more accessible. In the present context, the desired connotation is one of having achieved a certain quality, i.e. mastery. The term thus refers to an achieved state of consciousness.

vairagyam

As previously discussed, the word detachment can carry a connotation of aloofness, while non-attachment may easily be confused with an avoidance of both responsibility and commitment.

Vairagya, literally meaning "without color or passion", is translated here as dispassion. As noted in Sutra 1.12, the meaning of vairagya in this context is something akin to fervent equanimity.

Two esteemed traditional commentators say this of dispassion:

"....it is apparent that (the) non-attached yogi is always displeased with and free from desire for the enjoyable objects....(also) not envious of the enjoyers of those objects; and secondly he does not enjoy luxury on the lame excuse of desirelessness, as many people do." [53]

"The self restrained man who moves among objects with senses under the control of his own self, and free from affection and aversion, obtains tranquility. When there is tranquility there is an end of his miseries, for the mind of one of tranquil heart soon becomes steady." [54]

A Vedantic Perspective

"Desirelessness is wisdom. The two are not different; they are the same. Desirelessness is refraining from driving the mind toward any object. Wisdom means the appearances of no object. In other words, not seeking what is other than the Self is detachment or desirelessness; not leaving the Self is wisdom."

"All practices are followed only with the object of concentrating the mind. As all the mental activities like remembering, forgetting, desiring, hating, attracting, discarding, etc., are modifications of the mind, they cannot be one's true state. Simple, changeless being is one's true nature. Therefore, to know the truth of one's being and to be it is known as release from bondage ...until this state of tranquility of mind is firmly attained, the practice of unswerving abidance in the Self...is essential for an aspirant. (This practice) is not an effortless state of indolence... the act of communion with the Self, or remaining still inwardly, is intense activity which is performed with the entire mind and without break."

- excerpts from "The Spiritual Teaching of Ramana Maharshi" [55]

—— Exploration ——

Historically, the yoga sutras have been a clarion call to those who would ultimately wish to remove themselves from the continuous cycle of life, death and rebirth known as samsara. Granted, this is not likely the goal of the reader of these words, who is more likely to be concerned with being a better person or improving general quality of life. For many, if not most, the goal of being free from desire for objects seen or heard about would probably be an overreach. Nonetheless, the beauty of the yoga sutras is that they apply in principle regardless of one's individual life circumstances or one's life goals. It behooves us, then, to consider what our goals actually are, and to apply these guidelines accordingly.

With a good measure of self-reflection, together with sufficient motivation and a belief in the possibility of change, we may be able to achieve a significant degree of vairagya. When it occurs, this achievement is always evidenced by an increasing concordance between our actions, our emotional responses, and our consciously chosen ideals.

Patanjali has left us clues as to how to go about trying. The derivation of vasikara suggests a willful acquiescence, a mastery that is a kind of letting go.

Letting go of what? Letting go of the bond that tethers our emotions - the klista/aklista aspect of the vrittis - to the fulfillment of our personal desires. Letting go of the belief that any person, any thing, any power or accomplishment, or any rarefied state of mind can ultimately fulfill our deepest needs as human beings.

It may be worth revisiting the five klesas (the five root cases of suffering) as referenced in the discussion of klista- aklista in sutra 1.5. Once again, the klesas are:

1. avidya (ignorance of truth)
2. asmita (egoism, I-am-ness)
3. raga (attachment)
4. dvesa (aversion)
5. abhinivesa (longing for immortality).

Sir Monier Monier-Williams, the compiler of the Sanskrit English Dictionary which bears his name, offered an interesting insight into the meaning of samjna with "to cause to acquiesce". He notes that this phrase is "euphemistically said of a sacrificial victim, which ought not to be led forcibly to its death, but made to resign itself." [56]

The sacrificial victim here is none other than the personal ego-centered emotional life.

In considering sacrifice in the development of dispassion, it may be helpful to remember that the Latin root of sacrifice is sacere, meaning "to make sacred". In this sense a sacrifice is an offering, a relinquishment of a lesser value to a higher value that supersedes it.

Regarding obstacles to vairagya, whether we are stuck in trying to avoid that which is klista, or stuck in trying to attain that which is aklista, the principle remains the same.

—— **Further Reflections** ——

Dispassion is a quality which is easily claimed. The cultivation and consistent demonstration of dispassion, however, is a formidable task, even when attempted in only one small arena of one's life. Living one's life with true dispassion is perhaps the ultimate human challenge.

Traditionally, the journey to dispassion is seen as occurring in four distinct stages. These fours steps offer a description of what the aspirant can expect to encounter in his attempt to transform the nature of his own desires.

1. yatamana - awareness of striving
The first step is an acknowledgment that one's desires are problematic.

2. vyatireka - awareness of transgressions
The second step is the discernment of obstacles.

3. ekendriya: awareness of mind alone
The third step is when one's actions are successfully controlled, yet the mind remains attached to desires.

4. vasikara - awareness of mastery
The fourth step represents the willful acquiescence of personal desires and attachments.

Chapter 1, Sutra 16
—— Offering ——

You cannot force open the flower
of spiritual freedom.
It blooms on its own accord

- Vasant Lad, extract from "Strands of Eternity" [57]

1.16 tatparaṃ puruṣakhyātergunavaitṛṣnyam

tatparaṃ puruṣakhyātergunavaitṛṣnyam

Translations

tat (tad)	-	this
param	-	highest, lowest, most extreme
purusa	-	Self, the seer (see 1.3)
khyateh (here: discernment)	-	1. perception, knowledge 2. renown 3. declaration, assertion
from khya:	-	1. to make well known 2. to proclaim, to declare
(Continued)		

---

guna	-	1. one of three constituents of prakriti
		2. quality, property, attribute
		3. a single thread or strand
vaitrsnya	-	freedom from desire

1.16 The highest form of this, (arising from) discernment of Self (results in) freedom from desire for the gunas.

—— Introductory Remarks ——

This sutra continues the discussion of vairagya, indicating that there is an even higher level of dispassion than that defined in the previous sutra.

This highest level is defined as freedom from desire for even the basic constituents out of which objective and subjective worlds arise. This level of dispassion arises from the revelation, or discernment, of purusa or Self.

All four stages of dispassion as discussed in the previous sutra fall within the category of what is known as aparavairagya (non-transcendent dispassion). This sutra describes the transcendent level of dispassion known as paravairagya.

tatparam

Tatparam, meaning "the highest level of this" refers to vairagya.

purusa

Purusa refers to the Self, to pure consciousness or pure awareness.

In sutra 1.3, Patanjali used the term drstr (the seer) to refer to the Self. It is a more neutral term within the various schools of Indian thought, whereas the present usage of purusa requires more definitive explanations.

The Samkhya school posits that there are two distinct yet coexistent principles which constitute reality:

purusa - the Principle of Consciousness, Spirituality
prakriti - the Principle of Materiality or Matter

As Swami Veda Bharati (Usharbudh Arya) points out in his commentary, the term prakriti technically refers to unmanifest matter. By this definition prakriti is the subtle intangible origin of tangible matter (vikriti). Frequently, however, the term prakriti is used to refer to materiality in toto, both manifest and unmanifest. [58]

kyati

Kyati is translated variously as discernment, realization, and revelation. Purusa kyateh means the arising of wisdom evidenced by the growing ability to discern between purusa and prakriti, or Self and not-Self.

As the discernment of Self is usually a gradual process, purusa kyateh could conceivably refer to the entire process, from the initial stages of discrimination between Self and not-Self, up to the point of full unfailing recognition. In the context of the present discussion of transcendent dispassion it is fitting to relate purusa kyateh to the final stages of discernment of the Self.

guna

Guna is the Samkhya term for the attributes, or basic constituents, of prakriti. The gunas are three in number:

sattva - luminosity, clarity
rajas - activity, energy
tamas - inertia, darkness, dullness

As the sutra commentator Georg Feuerstein has stated very succinctly: "the gunas are not part of prakriti, the gunas **are** prakriti. They are the ultimate, irreducible building blocks of the material and mental world." [59]

According to Samkhya philosophy, the three gunas of prakriti exist in perfect equilibrium in their unmanifest state, but when that unmanifest potential is activated, there is a loss of equilibrium amongst the gunas.

vaitrsnya

In this sutra, Patanjali juxtaposes freedom from desire for objects of the everyday world or subtle celestial worlds, with freedom from desire for immersion even in the unmanifest aspects of materiality. He thereby draws attention to the radical difference between the these two levels of dispassion.

Immersion in unmanifest materiality may occur when, through intense meditation, the appearing objects of the world have been temporarily reduced back to their source and the yogi is able to contact and absorb himself in the gunas.

A more complete absorption in the gunas is said to occur in the process of cyclic rebirth or re-incarnation, between the time of death and rebirth. The highest level of dispassion occurs when the yogi finds even these absorptions wanting. It is important to remember that even though broad potentials of meditative practice are being described here, the practitioner should always stay grounded in the truth of one's actual present condition.

Patanjali reminds us that freedom from desire for the gunas arises as a result of the realization of purusa (Self).

In the words of Swami Veda Bharati: "It is the revelation of the spiritual principle that leads to the absence of thirst, rather than the absence of thirst leading to this revelation ." [60]

A Perspective From Two Yogis

Swami Hariharananda Aranya, in his commentary on the yoga sutras, describes what occurs when the yogi fails to achieve realization of purusa. This explanation introduces the term 'buddhi,' which in the scheme of Samkhya is the faculty of intelligence and intuitive wisdom, the most subtle and pure manifestation of the gunas: [61]

"After withdrawing the mind from objects through Vasikara, concentration in an arrested state of the mind through the knowledge about Purusa has to be practised. When the knowledge of the nature of Purusa dawns, the mind becomes free from thoughts of worldly objects, and is only occupied with matters relating to discrimination. Those who withdraw their minds from external objects by detachment (Vasikara) and concentrate on the unmanifested or the void as the final principle not noticing at the same time the distinction between Purusa and 'Buddhi'

(Continued)

are not on the right path. Since they have failed to discover the distinction between Purusa and 'Buddhi,' their state of concentration is not complete and does not bring them towards the final state of 'Nirodha' or ultimate dissolution of the mind."]

From Swami Veda Bharati's sutra commentary: [62]

"When knowledge of the nature of Purusa is acquired, then there is no more inclination in the satisfied mind to be engrossed in the unmanifested Prakriti or the void; on the other hand, (there) develops a desire to engage...in the contemplation of the Purusa principle and thus get perpetual peace."

"A complete separation from the Gunas and their mutations then arises. Paravairagya or the highest detachment and unadulterated knowledge of the purusa-principle are inseparable. Only by that means...liberation, in the shape of complete cessation of the mind, is attainable."

——— **Exploration** ———

Patanjali is speaking here about an ultimate level of dispassion. The paravairagya which proceeds from revelation of the Self is none other than liberation from material existence.

Sutras such as this, which deal with transcendent states of a very high order, may be easily grasped at a conceptual level, but true experiential realization is a different matter entirely. Nevertheless, a conceptual understanding may aid in developing the discernment which drives our spiritual growth.

To recap the comparison between this sutra and the previous one, we see that dispassion falls into two broad categories:

1. Aparavairagya. Dispassion for all objects, gross or subtle, seen or heard about. This dispassion is known as non-transcendent dispassion because this extraordinary achievement still does not free the yogi from his attachment to material existence.

2. Paravairagya. Dispassion for even the gunas. This is known as transcendent dispassion. When the yogi finally achieves dispassion for even the gunas, he is completely released from his attachment to material existence.

Patanjali raises the important point that it is realization or discernment of the Self that brings about the state of transcendent dispassion. Freedom for the yogi lies in the ability to recognize and cling to that which is eternally true. Without this recognition and the ability to discern between the relative truths and impermanent achievements of the material plane and the ultimate truth of the Spiritual Self, transcendent dispassion cannot take hold.

Continuous unbroken discernment between purusa and prakriti and total dispassion towards the world of materiality, manifest as the final stages of spiritual transformation.

Amongst commentators there is, understandably, a great deal of disagreement as to the precise conditions of the yogi who is approaching or has achieved paravairagya.

There is also a great deal of disagreement as to the status of the yogi who mistakes immersion in the gunas for true liberation. These disparities reflect some of the basic differences between Buddhist and yoga traditions in regards to how the nature of purusa or Self is perceived (as shall be seen in the discussion of Sutra 1.17).

In the meantime, it is undoubtedly safe to assume that the reader has at least a few object-oriented desires with which to deal. In keeping with this simple truth, it is would be wise to maintain a focus on issues that are real within our present context.

Trevor Leggett's comments on vairagya, the gunas, and vision of the Self are excellent in this regard, as they elucidate how our states of mind are affected by the gunas.

"Even a glimpse of the Self frees from many long-standing obsessions. They are not exactly conquered triumphantly; they simply lose their importance because they become illusory...Take the guna rajas - passion-struggle. Normally this is felt as the fight for success in a particular thing; that thing is the object of attachment, and joy is hoped for when it is attained. But a man whose attachment is for rajas itself does not mind much what thing it is that he fights for. His joy is in the struggle, and when he is successful he is rather indifferent to the object. It was merely a field for his rajas. Such men are mountaineers in everything. It is not that there is anything at the top of the mountain; they simply wish to 'conquer' it, as they put it. In the world they are often magnanimous to those whom they have defeated; it is victory itself that they want, not any particular success. Other people, traveling in the wake of such conquerors, may reap benefits, but the heroes themselves frequently waste their lives." "In the same way a man can be attached to the lethargy of tamas, which gives him a cheerful indifference to everything; or the serenity and clarity of the individual self in sattva, which he does not wish to break up in favour of expansion into the unknown depths of the real Self." [63]

——— **Further Reflections** ———

The following expansion upon an ancient celestial analogy will perhaps illuminate the nature of the relationship between purusa, buddhi (the most purified level of mind), and the vrittis (normal activities of the mind).

Purusa is like the sun. The sun is a star, and stars are self-luminous, lending their light to whatever and whoever is nearby. It is through the light of our sun that life as we know it on earth is supported.

The human mindfield may be likened to the earth, for the earth is completely dependent upon the sun (purusa) not only for its light, but for the place it occupies in the heavens.

Our individual minds may be likened to the specific places we inhabit on the earth. From our individual vantage points, we are only able to see the sun directly as long as there are no obstructions. This may occur when two conditions are met: when the face of the earth on which "I" stand is turned towards the sun, and when "I" look from under a cloudless sky with nothing obstructing my view.

My unobstructed view of the sun from my vantage point on the earth may be likened to buddhi (the highest level of purified mind).

Finally, the moon may be likened to the vrittis. Neither the earth (the mindfield) nor the moon (the activities of the mind) are self-luminous or self-sustaining. But because of the nature of the moon's orbit, it has the capacity to reflect the light of the sun into the darkness of earth's night.

In truth, when the face of the earth where "I" stand is turned away from the sun, it is the "light of the moon" that lights my path.

May that light gently guide me ever towards its source.

Chapter 1, Sutra 17
—— Offering ——

I Am: yet what I am none cares or knows...
I am the self-consumer of my woes –
They rise and vanish in oblivious host
And yet I am...

- John Clare, extract from "I Am" [64]

1.17 vitarkavicārānandāsmitārūpānugamāt
saṃprajñātaḥ

vitarkavicārānandāsmitārūpānugamātsaṃprajñātaḥ

Translations

vitarka (here: conjecture)	-	1. reasoning, speculation 2. thought with verbal associations
from tarka:	-	reasoning, philosophical inquiry
vicara (here: subtilization)	-	1. reflection, contemplation, intuition 2. thought with few verbal associations

(Continued)

from cara:	-	1. to move through, pervade 2. to spread out, expand, be diffused 3. self-locomotion
ananda	-	bliss, joy, beatitude
asmita	-	"I-am-ness"
rupa	-	form
anugamat (here: proceeds successively)	-	1. following after (in life or death) 2. entering into, approaching 3. dying out, being extinguished
samprajnatah (here: cognitive samadhi)	-	1. perfect integrated knowledge 2. discerned, known accurately

1.17 Cognitive samadhi proceeds successively (through) conjecture, subtilization, bliss, and the "I am" form.

—— Introductory Remarks ——

This sutra goes on to define four levels of samprajnata (cognitive samadhi) which correlate with the attainments of non-transcendent dispassion.

Samadhi is defined here (in advance of the formal introduction of the term in sutra 1.20) as a deep meditative absorption. Samprajnata samadhi is said to be **cognitive** samadhi as it has some aspect of materiality as its support.

According to this sutra, samprajnata samadhi in its full scope proceeds progressively through four distinct levels.

Commentators vary in their understanding of the characteristics of these four levels, but despite the many differences there
is a general consensus on at least three points:

1. The four levels represent increasingly subtle levels of mind.

2. Generally speaking, each level manifests itself as the
processes of the mind in the previous level are attenuated.

3. The four levels cover the full spectrum of cognitive
samadhi.

vitarka

Vitarka is usually translated as "applied thought", "with
reasoning" or "with verbal associations". Here it is translated as
"conjecture" and implies a concrete level of the activities of the
mind as they relate to the object of meditation.

It is not the object of meditation which defines vitarka but
rather the nature of the attention brought to bear upon that
object. The concretized thought processes in vitarka, and the
ensuing effects of that on the entire energy field of the practitioner,
suggests a correlation with the tamas guna.

vicara

Vicara represents a movement from the gross towards
the subtle. As the attention of the mind shifts from the gross
to the subtle there is a concomitant shift in the mind's mode
of operation and also, as noted above, upon the entire energy
field of the practitioner. The normal verbal thought processes
are attenuated, giving way to a more intuitive, contemplative,
non-verbal modality.

The root cara and its various meanings taken as a whole
suggest a correlation with the rajas guna.

ananda

Ananda is a feeling of bliss, ecstasy, or beatitude. In samadhi with ananda the mind is turned back onto its own inherent qualities. Bliss is an inherent aspect of the purified mind, and the dropping away of vitarka and vicara unveils this ever-present potential.

In ananda accompanied samadhi we may see a correlation with the sattva guna.

asmita

Asmita means "I-am-ness". When even the feeling of bliss in the purified mind has been quieted, the mind is able to affix solely on the "I am" realization. Asmita represents the highest level of cognitive samadhi, yet it is still equated with sarupya, the misidentification with the citta vritti.

Asmita accompanied samadhi is a transcendence of the attachments of vitarka, vicara and ananda, but the full realization of purusa is not yet achieved.

rupa

Rupa means form. Some texts on the yoga sutras do not include the term rupa here. On occasions when it does form part of the text, it is usually taken to refer to asmita, the last of the four levels. In this way the term rupa serves as a reminder that even though samadhi with asmita is the most subtle level of samprajnata, it nonetheless has a subtle level of cognitive support and remains in the realm of cognitive samadhi.

There is also an historical implication of the use of the term rupa here, which provides valuable insight (see comments below).

anugamat

Anugamat is usually translated as "accompanied by". Here it means accompanied by vitarka, vicara, ananda or asmita. These four levels normally occur in the order shown, with each successive level being unveiled as the prior level is superceded.

samprajnata

Prajna is translated as wisdom. Samprajnata samadhi may be rendered as "wisdom meditation", otherwise known as cognitive samadhi.

——— Exploration ———

The four levels of samprajnata samadhi are said to be cognitive as they are levels of meditation supported by the cognition of some object, knowledge or experience. All four levels of cognitive samadhi correlate with the state of non-transcendent dispassion.

In samprajnata samadhi the yogi is able to ascertain with clarity, and in progressively subtle levels, the true nature of an object, though it is only the **material nature** of the object that is ascertainable at this level of meditation. In order to fully ascertain the true spiritual nature inherent within an object, one must have first achieved the discernment of purusa from which transcendent dispassion arises.

The following excerpt is from Swami Veda Bharati's commentary:

"The mind, an evolute of unconscious matter, has no capability to grasp the pure consciousness principle. Even a semblance of such grasping does not begin until asmita is realized....What then is the purpose of such realization at these various levels in samprajnata samadhi? They are to fulfill the purpose described in [sutras] 1.15,16: to develop dispassion towards each level...At each level one feels that the next subtler level is purer. But upon examination by realization it is found that the purity is only relative..." [65]

Let us consider how samadhi accompanied by vitarka, vicara, ananda and asmita might be described within this framework.

Samadhi accompanied by vitarka may be described as a meditative state in which the ordinary activities of the mind have been slowed down or quieted. In such a state one might have a realization in regards to specific attributes of an object of meditation.

A deep samadhi with vitarka may produce an experiential knowingness of the object that penetrates beyond its "normal" reality. If the object of meditation is the mind itself, this experience may entail a profound encounter with the reality of the discursive, dichotomizing mind.

Samadhi accompanied by vicara might involve a further quieting of the mind, perhaps with a realization of some very subtle truth about the object of meditation that had previously been unreachable.

A deep samadhi with vicara might produce such a vivid "non-ordinary" view of the object that it's so-called normal reality is seriously challenged. If the object of meditation is the mind itself, the experience may entail a direct encounter with the non-discursive, non-dichotomizing aspects of mind.

Moving on to ananda, samadhi accompanied by ananda might produce an in-depth understanding of the dual nature of the pleasure-pain mechanism within the mind.

A deep samadhi with ananda might be experienced as an

unequivocal affirmation that joy is man's potential heritage. This could be seen as a temporary transcendence of the klista/aklista aspects of the vrittis. If the object of meditation is the mind itself, one may realize that the nature of the purified mind is bliss.

The fourth level of samadhi accompanied by asmita (I-am-ness) is a rarefied and highly focused state that very likely will reveal its own meaning. The experience may be registered as an entrance into a profound knowingness of not just "I am not my body" but "I am not my mind".

It is said that the "I am" state is the original seed of individuation from which the personal self evolved outward into manifestation.

When the "I am" realization occurs in samadhi, the mind is concentrated in the inward turned face of buddhi. Buddhi, as noted in the discussion of sutra 1.16, is "purified mind". It is the first evolute of prakriti and the most subtle and pure manifestation of the gunas, and is thus the most pure aspect of the entire mindfield.

It is in this state that the yogi is able to make the initial recognition, through direct experience, that the source of his awareness is not within buddhi but rather that buddhi is simply the receiver of the light of purusa.

Samadhi with the "I am" realization is the gateway within the mind between the outward path to the realm of Matter and the inward path to the realm of Spirit. It is this state of consciousness which most closely approximates the balanced equilibrium of the gunas which exists in unmanifest prakriti.

Now, regarding the term rupa in this sutra, there was an ancient classification of the levels of meditative absorption which is believed to have existed prior to the time of the Buddha. This ancient system was an eightfold classification which distinguished rupa from arupa absorptions and which to this day remains the framework of Buddhist teachings.

Within this ancient eightfold description are two contrasting fields of meditative absorption, each comprised of four levels. The first are known as rupa-jhana, meaning that they appear in relation to the Sphere of Form. The second set are known as arupa-jhana, and appear in relation to the Sphere of Formlessness. The following is a comparison of the four rupa-jhana absorptions and Patanjali's four levels of samprajnata samadhi.

<u>Four Rupa-jhanaAbsorptions</u> (Pali rather than Sanskrit)

1st level   Vitakka (initial application of the mind)
            Vicara (sustained attention to the object)
2nd level Piti (joy)
3rd level Sukha (blissful equanimity)
4th level Ekaggata (one-pointed mindfulness)

Comparing samprajnata with the rupa-jhana system, the major differences are as follows:

1. Vitakka and vicara are coupled together in the first level and given slightly different meanings.

2. In the second and third level piti takes the place of vicara, in effect expanding the ananda level into a two-step process of piti and sukha.

3. In the fourth level, ekaggata, which may be defined as an ultimate one-pointed concentration of the mind, replaces asmita.

———— **Further Reflections** ————

This sutra is a road map to meditative absorption, one which Patanjali presents using the language of experience, not that of intellectual analysis. Yet this very same sutra tends to elicit commentaries of a very complex and analytical nature, the present study notwithstanding.

Why is this so? Perhaps it is inevitable that abstract intellectual analysis becomes the primary mode to express what lies outside of commonly understood experience.

Examined collectively these intellectual analyses may appear as conflicting maps. But all the complex and detailed systematic explanations are really just personal annotations on the map of human consciousness. They are meant to be useful, but if they do not serve to help us pierce through the layers of intellectual grasping to the heart of the matter, then it might be best to set them aside.

The classifications of samadhi in this sutra are only descriptive. They describe possibilities that are inherent within the mind. They should not be taken as prescriptive. But no matter how well we understand this, there is always the danger, as with all road maps of the psyche, that the descriptions on the map may stand in the way of one's own authentic experience.

Rigorously honest self-reflection is essential in developing discernment, for each level of samadhi can only be visited with the level of understanding which one actually brings to the experience, and there is a vast terrain that lies between momentary realizations, even profound ones, and stabilized states of awareness.

At a simple practical level, the progressive levels of cognitive samadhi may be seen as analogous to an increasingly challenging asana or pranayama practice, wherein a practitioner may or may not be able to achieve a specified form in its full perfection.

Indeed, it is not the purpose of an idealized form to measure one's abilities. Rather, the principles embodied in the form should be applied to the individual in appropriate and realistic ways, depending upon that individual's actual needs.

Sutra - 17

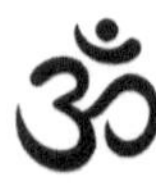

Chapter 1, Sutra 18
—— *Offering* ——

Scattered with so much going on inside,
I long for nothing but an inner unity.

- Jalal Al-Din Rumi [66]

1.18 virāmapratyayābhyāsapūrvaḥ
saṃskāraśeṣo 'nyaḥ

virāmapratyayābhyāsapūrvaḥ saṃskāraśeṣo'nyaḥ

<table>
<tr><td colspan="3"><h2>Translations</h2></td></tr>
<tr><td>virama</td><td>-</td><td>1. cessation, termination
2. to come to an end or rest
3. desistance, abstention from</td></tr>
<tr><td>pratyaya</td><td>-</td><td>seed-cognition (see 1.10)</td></tr>
<tr><td>abhyasa</td><td>-</td><td>practice (see 1.12)</td></tr>
<tr><td>purvah</td><td>-</td><td>1. being before or in front of, first
2. preceded by, accompanied by</td></tr>
<tr><td>samskara -
(here: habitual
potency)</td><td></td><td>1. mental impression from past actions
2. making ready, purification
3. a purificatory ceremony or ritual</td></tr>
<tr><td>(Continued)</td><td></td><td></td></tr>
</table>

seso	-	1. remainder, that which is left
		2. residue, remnant
		3. end, conclusion, result
anyah	-	other

1.18 The other (a-cognitive samadhi), being preceded (only) by practice of the seed-cognition of cessation, has that habitual potency as residue.

—— Introductory Remarks ——

This sutra tells us that in addition to cognitive samadhi there is also another type of samadhi known as a-cognitive samadhi (asamprajnata).

This other samadhi is defined as a state which follows upon the practice of virama pratyaya. Having been preceded only by this practice, it is only the samskaras of this practice which remain active in a-cognitive samadhi.

virama

Virama is usually translated as cessation. To get a clearer picture of the meaning of virama, let us contrast virama with nirodha, which is also translated as cessation.

Nirodha in relation to the citta vritti has a connotation of harnessing, control, restraint, confining or turning back, and is being viewed in this study as referring to the entire process of controlling the citta vritti, from beginning to end. Virama, on the other hand, connotes termination.

Termination of what? Traditionally there have been two

basic streams of answers to this question, and these two streams have led to controversy as to the precise nature of a-cognitive samadhi.

The first view claims that virama refers to termination of the citta vritti themselves, that is, termination of the normal processes of the mind and their associated conditions. The second view claims that virama refers to termination of identification with the citta vritti, thus robbing the citta vritti of their potency.

This second view is founded upon the idea that the most basic component of the ordinary processes of mind is self-identification, stemming from the commingling within the mind of primordial non-objective awareness (the seer) and the movements of the mind associated with objective awareness. It is asserted that when this most basic identification with the ordinary processes of the mind ceases, the other processes of the mind, though they do not necessarily cease, are transformed in a way that makes them no longer binding.

pratyaya

The term pratyaya is commonly translated as cognitive cause. The translation given here is seed-cognition (see comments sutra 1.10).

In the same way that the vritti of dreamless sleep was shown to be dependent upon abhava pratyaya (the seed-cognition of absence of the other vrittis), the indication here is that the objective support for the mind in virama pratyaya abhyasa is the seed-cognition of cessation or termination.

abhyasa

Abhyasa means practice, indicating that Patanjali is referring to virama pratyaya as a practice.

Patanjali defined practice in sutra 1.13 as "the willful effort towards steadiness in that (nirodha)." This broad definition serves as an umbrella for the many possible forms of practice which contribute to nirodha, from the beginning of the process of controlling the citta vritti to its final fruition.

The practice of virama pratyaya, however, refers to a very specific and advanced meditative practice in which the only "object" is the seed-cognition of cessation.

purvah

Purvah, preceded by, is descriptive of anya - the other (a-cognitive samadhi) - indicating that it is preceded by the practice of the seed-cognition of cessation.

samskara

The verbal root kr means to do or to act. Sam has the meaning of complete, altogether, perfect. Samskara is translated here as habitual potency.

sesa

Sesa means residue, remainder, or that which is left over when something has been removed or dissolved.

It would seem remiss to not mention here that as a proper noun Sesa is also the name of the mythological thousand-headed serpent identified with Wisdom. This thousand-headed serpent is a symbol of eternity, which in Hinduism is sometimes represented as providing both the couch and a protective umbrella for the god Vishnu. Another name for this Sesa, the King of the Serpents, is Adisesa, "who descended in the form of Patanjali and gave us the yoga darsana."

anya

Anya means other, that which is other than, or which lies beyond the previous subject (samprajnata samadhi). Anya refers to asamprajnata or a-cognitive samadhi, a transcendent state of awareness which yields neither to words nor mental concepts.

A Traditional Parable

There was a child made all of salt who very much wanted to know where he had come from. So he set out on a long journey and traveled to many lands in pursuit of this understanding. Finally, he came to the shore of the great ocean. How marvelous, he cried, and stuck one foot in the water. The ocean beckoned him in further, saying 'If you wish to know who you are, do not be afraid.' The salt child walked further and further into the water, dissolving with each step, and at the end exclaimed 'Ah, now I know who I am.'

—— Exploration ——

A-cognitive samadhi may be preceded by the practice of virama pratyaya, the seed-cognition of cessation, as a bridge between the highest level of cognitive samadhi (accompanied by asmita) and a-cognitive samadhi. However, as we shall see in sutras 1.19 and 1.20, it is not the only practice to serve this purpose.

Through the progressive attenuation of the normal processes of the mind represented by the four levels of cognitive samadhi, the mind becomes increasingly disentangled from its habitual modalities. But attenuation is like repeatedly cutting a piece of pie in half - a process which can never, no matter how long it is repeated, produce a complete absence of pie.

In the fourth and last stage of cognitive samadhi, in which "I am" is the only remaining object in one's meditation, a state of mind exists which is very far removed from the ordinary daily activities of the mind. Still, this last stage of samadhi must be transformed before the transcendent state of a-cognitive samadhi makes its appearance.

Swami Veda Bharati, made the following comment:

"The practice of virama-pratyaya means constantly, repeatedly, entering into that awareness [virama- pratyaya]. The process of virama-pratyaya-abhyasa is establishing it again and again into the mindfield. It is brought to perfection when even the vritti "I am" from asmita is abandoned." [67]

When one enters a-cognitive samadhi through the practice of virama pratyaya, there is a mark of the virama practice left upon the mind as a residue. Patanjali calls this mark sesa samskara.

Traditionally, samskara has two streams of meaning:

1. An impression, latent impression, or habitual potency within the mind which results from past experiences or past actions, or the total accumulation of such impressions or potencies;

2. A cleansing, purificatory, or transformative ritual, such as a rite of passage.

At first glance these two meanings may seem antithetical. But if we consider that the purpose of rituals such as rites of passage is to create an atmosphere in which deep and lasting impressions can be imprinted upon the minds of participants, the connection becomes clear.

An interesting thing about the mind's inner landscape of samskaras is that it is constantly being remodeled. That means that while we are highly susceptible to changing circumstances in our lives, we also have a tremendous capacity for change.

Yet there is no generic formula for intentionally producing desired change. Thus have arisen the many and varied ceremonies, rituals and traditions of society, whose purpose is to leave something as close to an indelible mark upon the mind as is possible. In this way an intentional samskara is produced which may in time overshadow previously embedded samskaras inclined towards a different course.

In relation to the yoga sutras, samskara is nearly always defined within the first stream of meaning. In the words of Fernando Tola and Carmen Dragonetti:

"These latent subliminal impressions constitute the predisposition, the "seed" of other new manifestations of mental life; they rest in what may be called the unconsciousness in a potential form and will necessarily (eventually) actualize themselves..." [68]

Ian Whicher, in his sutra commentary, briefly points to the second stream of meaning, then goes on to discuss the more general definition of samskara as impression:

"In Hindu tradition samskaras can refer to the rites of passage such as birth rites (jatakarma), marriage rites (vivaha), and death rites (antyesti), rites that are all intended to purify and transform the individual at specific phases of life"...

..."Pertaining to the individual person, samskaras are responsible for the production of various psychomental phenomena...the (samskaras) have internal currents or a "flow" of their own, currents that clearly influence or effect a person's intentional and volitional nature. When certain impressions, through the repeated practice of certain actions or by constant addition of like-impressions, become strong enough, the propensities they create impel a person in a certain direction." [69]

------ **Further Reflections** ------

The eightfold rupa and arupa stages of meditation are listed below. Included are four **rupa** stages (with form) and four **arupa** stages (without form), correlating with cognitive and a-cognitve samadhi.

Once again, it should be noted that the four rupa stages are identified in a slightly different manner by Patanjali in sutra 1.17. The arupa stages remain unnamed in the yoga sutras. The following breakdown is ancient in origin but is still used today in traditional Buddhist teachings.

<u>Four Rupa-jhana Absorptions</u> (terms are Pali)
1st level   Vitakka (initial application of the mind)
             Vicara (sustained attention to the object)
2nd level Piti (joy)
3rd level   Sukha (blissful equanimity)
4th level   Ekaggata (one-pointed mindfulness)

<u>Four A-rupa-jhana Absorptions</u> (Buddhist teachings)
1st level   Dimension of Infinite Space
2nd level Dimension of Infinite Consciousness
3rd level   Dimension of Nothingness
4th level   Dimension of Neither Perception nor
             Non-Perception

It may also be worth noting that it is at the level of asmita that a fundamental controversy exists within some yoga schools of thought. Samadhi accompanied by asmita is generally viewed as the level of meditation in which the practitioner is able to directly perceive, in an experiential way, the core from which his individuality arises. This realization is termed the "I am" state.

This "I am" realization is not considered to be the ultimate level of samadhi. Rather it is simply the most purified level of mind which manifests in cognitive samadhi. In Patanjali's yoga sutras, it is explicit in the presentation of a-cognitive samadhi that all four levels of samprajnata have been attenuated before the a-cognitive state appears.

Yet some traditional streams of thought have taken the position that asmita is a manifestation of a-cognitive samadhi, resulting in the conclusion that the "I am" realization represents the pinnacle of human achievement in the realm of consciousness. This is not Patanjali's position.

Chapter 1, Sutra 19
—— Offering ——

Little lamb, who made thee?
Dost thou know who made thee?
Little lamb, I'll tell thee...
He is called by thy name,
For He calls Himself a Lamb.
He is meek, and He is mild,
He became a little child.
I a child, and thou a lamb,
We are called by His name...

- William Blake, extract from "The Lamb" [70]

1.19 bhavapratyayo videhaprakṛtilayānām

bhavapratyayo videhaprakṛtilayānām

Translations

bhava	-	being, becoming
pratyaya	-	seed-cognition (see 1.10 and 1.18)
videha	-	bodiless, discarnate
prakriti	-	the Principle of Materiality (see 1.16 under purusa and guna)
layanam	-	absorption in

1.19 Those who are bodiless or absorbed in prakriti (rest upon) the seed-cognition of becoming.

—— Introductory Remarks ——

This sutra juxtaposes the practice of bhava pratyaya with the practice of virama pratyaya, contrasting the **sesa samskaras** or latent impressions which result from the two practices. Specifically mentioned are two classes of beings who have attained a non-ordinary state of existence via bhava pratyaya - the videhas and the prakritilayas - but this is not to say that they are the only practitioners on this path.

bhava pratyaya

Many commentators on this sutra have presented bhava pratyaya as meaning "caused by birth" or "resulting from birth". This is a very common translation of the Sanskrit text. However, in this context there is a contrary meaning attached to pratyaya in sutras 1.10, 1.18 and 1.20, where pratyaya is an active process related to the mental content that determines states of consciousness. In the yoga sutras, pratyaya means cognitive support, cognitive cause, or as translated here "seed-cognition", and is an integral part of Patanjali's presentation of meditative practice as a means of spiritual transformation.

The literal meaning of bhava is being or becoming. In keeping with the contextual meaning of pratyaya as the cognitive support or seed-cognition in meditation, bhava pratyaya is rendered here as "seed-cognition of becoming". This connotes a pratyaya based upon an intentional merging of one's consciousness in devotional practice, as presented in the yoga sutras as one of the primary paths of meditative practice.

As for the more common translation of bhava pratyaya as "caused by birth", there is a certain irony in saying that the condition of those who are disembodied - the videhas and prakritilayas - is caused by birth.

In a devotional practice, one identifies with some being or consciousness outside of one's current self-identification. The choice of object in a meditative practice of "merging" in this way is of paramount importance. Historically, there have been numerous established meditative practices of merging one's consciousness not only with God, but also with gods and demigods as well as personifications of forces and subtle elements in nature.

videha

Videha means bodiless, without form. This refers to beings who, no longer identified with the physical body, have abandoned the body yet still maintain a celestial form comprised of the subtlest levels of mind and ego. They are sometimes called the "bodiless shining gods". Patanjali does not address the issue of whether videhas disassociate from their physical form before or after death.

prakriti layanam

Prakriti layanam means merged in prakriti. It refers to those whose intellect has been resolved into the material cause in Nature, having abandoned the evolutes of prakriti. The implication is that they have merged their consciousness with such material cause in Nature, as opposed to merging with a higher consciousness.

On Videha-Mukti

He alone is Videha Mukta who has become the Supreme being and whose Atman is enjoying everlasting peace and perpetual bliss. One who finds his Atman in everything and everything in his Atman is Videha Mukta. One who realizes the nature of Atman is Videha Mukta....(and) has no bondage. Aham Brahmasmi, I am absolute consciousness only. [71]

- Tejo Bindu Upanishad

—— Exploration ——

This sutra mentions two unique categories of beings and its precise meaning will likely remain in question. The implication seems to be that the states of existence of the videhas and the prakritilayas is a natural outcome of their practice of bhava pratyaya.

Perhaps there is a cautionary note here regarding a practitioner's choice of object. If one engages in a practice of the seed cognition of becoming or merging one's consciousness with the object of meditation, then one should choose carefully the object of one's devotion and practice with the end result in mind.

If the subject of one's practice is a subtle element or material cause of prakriti, then one might ultimately reach the state of existence of a prakritilaya. Likewise, a practice devoted to merging one's consciousness with celestial beings or gods might lead to such a celestial realm.

Some commentators have proclaimed that the videhas and prakritilayas believe "mistakenly" that they have achieved the final goal of yoga when in fact they have not, though this does not appear to be an assumption that Patanjali himself intended.

It is probably advisable to exercise caution when painting with broad strokes in regards to the intentions or "mistakes" of entire classes of beings. After all, perhaps these rarefied beings do what they do for a reason, such as service to others, in the manner of a Bodhisattva.

The yoga sutras are a presentation of the potentialities of human consciousness. The reader is reminded that the most potent application of the concepts and prescripts offered here will be one that recognizes the actual condition and needs of the individual. While an understanding of general potentialities can help us form an appropriate framework for reaching our full potential as individuals, this requires an honest and insightful assessment of what will best serve both our immediate and long term goals.

——— Further Reflections ———

From a historical perspective, there is another long-standing controversy hinted at by this sutra. Some Buddhist schools of thought as well as some Vedantic traditions have concluded that Hindu and Samkhya based yoga schools have incorrectly subscribed to the notion of a permanent and irreducible individualized self, whereas in Buddhism and Vedanta, it is the realization of the fundamental non-reality of the individualized self that supports its other tenets.

But even though certain historical figures in yoga certainly did posit the existence of an eternal individualized self, there is nothing in Patanjali's presentation of the yoga sutras to support such a notion.

Even in the fourth chapter of the yoga sutras, where Patanjali takes up this discussion at a deeper level, it may be seen that such arguments against Buddhist and Vedantic philosophy are actually arguments initiated within the yoga commentarial tradition, not by Patanjali himself.

Comparing philosophical and religious systems gives us an opportunity to appreciate the fact that actual experience is the basis for both, but the expression of that actual experience is necessarily shaped by the language and thought patterns of the mind or minds in which the experience is rooted. This serves as a profound reminder that in order to grasp innate potentials of the human mind with clarity, we must be able to see beyond sociological context.

In the words of a contemporary Tibetan Buddhist teacher:

"The teachings of all tenet systems on ultimate truth conceals its meaning. The pure truth, that is, the ultimate truth, is obscured by every system of tenets. The ultimate truth of reality, the truth beyond all illusion, is not something to be found in words and concepts. In fact, the ultimate truth is precisely that which is beyond all conceptual processes. Praising one's own views, belittling the views of others, grandly proclaiming the meaning of emptiness, of existence, non-existence, and so forth are all modes of mental grasping, of intellectual harispication that obscure the sun of ultimate truth with the clouds of verbal debate, formalistic logic and scriptural citations."

"It is because ultimate truth is profound and complex that one needs extensive learning to begin to appreciate it. Because of its ultimacy, its realization requires deep integrative contemplation and the entrance into profound meditative states. It is realized only in the direct yogic perception of [a practitioner] within his/her meditative state. It can never be realized by ordinary worldly meditations as it transcends them all." [72]

Chapter 1, Sutra 20
—— Offering ——

Courage is the spirit that places you
on top of the mountain
When it's easier to never leave the ground

- Anonymous

1.20 śraddhāvīryasmṛtisamādhiprajñāpūrvaka
itareṣām

śraddhāvīryasmṛtisamādhiprajñāpūrvaka itareṣām

Translations

sraddha	-	1. faith, conviction, belief in 2. trust, confidence
virya	-	1. strength, energy, vigor 2. valor
smrti	-	1. memory, remembrance, 2. mindfulness, presence of mind
samadhi (here: untranslated)	-	1. meditation, contemplation 2. intense absorption of mind, as in meditation or prayer
(Continued)		

prajna	-	wisdom, intuitive wisdom, highest knowledge
purvaka	-	preceded by
itaresam	-	of the others

1.20 Conviction, inner strength, mindfulness, samadhi, and samadhi-wisdom precedes (the accomplishment of) the others

—— Introductory Remarks ——

This sutra further contrasts virama pratyaya and the bhava pratyaya of the videhas and prakritilayas with the approach of others who practice what is traditionally known as upaya pratyaya, upaya meaning "skillful means".

virama pratyaya: seed-cognition of cessation 1.18
bhava pratyaya: seed-cognition of being/becoming 1.19
upaya pratyaya: seed-cognition of skillful means 1.20

In accordance with historical tradition, Patanjali lists the five factors of upaya pratyaya as faith, inner strength, memory, samadhi and the wisdom derived from samadhi.

sraddha

According to Sir Monier Monier-Williams, sraddha (derived from srat or srad) is believed to be related to satya (truth, faithfulness) and probably allied to the English words heart and hearten through the Latin root cor or cord (creed, credo). [73]

Translated here as conviction, sraddha might be likened to "belief of the heart" or perhaps "belief which heartens".

Some commentators discuss sraddha as faith in God. Some speak of faith in the process of yoga. Some speak of the necessity of confidence in the teacher and confidence in oneself.

Ian Whicher, in his yoga sutra commentary, presents the following discussion:

"On the path of Yoga one places one's faith in the presence or awareness of purusa, which is without qualities or properties and yet is the authentic foundation of one's existence. Yoga does not call for mere blind faith but stresses the need for clarity of mind initially grounded in the direct experience of sattva–which, as Vyasa asserts: "like a good mother protects the yogin." When purusa is perceived as being distinct from the extrinsic (gunic) identity of self–however sattvic–which lays claim to the experience in the form of "my knowledge," "my reward", "my experience," the yogin then loses interest in any attachment to the things of the mind; the personality is purified and relinquishes all claim to authentic identity..." [74]

Sraddha implies here not just any quality of faith, but the calm and abiding conviction which comes from well-founded trust.

virya

Whereas sraddha is a feminine term, virya is a masculine term relating to vigor or virility. It is translated here as inner strength, the kind which makes commitment and perseverance possible. Virya is usually related to the energy that is necessary to sustain one's efforts.

Swami Hariharananda Aranya states:

"When the mind is tired and wants to drift to a different subject, the power which can bring it back to devotional practice is called Virya....it is implied that the Sraddha and

Virya mentioned here relate to the means for attainment of Kaivalya...There may be Sraddha and Virya for other objects but they do not bring about Yoga or the state of liberation." [75]

Gary Kraftsow has described the relationship between sraddha and virya as follows:

"Virya relates to where we put our attention, and where we put our attention has to do with our conditioning and is connected with our desires and motivations. Unless we have a deep faith or confidence or certainty, we can't simply choose to direct our attention to God. It's a nice idea, but it takes a tremendous amount of energy to be able to do that and override your past conditioning. So there has to be some deep faith in order to direct one's attention." [76]

smriti

Smriti was introduced in sutra 1.11 as memory, one of the five normal processes of the mind.

Here smriti connotes mindfulness of the path, the goal and the means. This evolution from memory to mindfulness represents nothing less than the transformation of memory in service of practice.

According to Swami Veda Bharati:

"The fivefold method of this sutra is identical to the Buddhist tradition of cultivating five strengths, among which smriti (sati in Pali) is the most important. Practicing mindfulness... is perhaps the most central part of Buddhist meditation practice. Thus it appears that the true meaning of the word smriti as it occurs in this sutra is preserved in the Buddhist practice of sati-patthana, a mindfulness that is maintained not only on one's meditation seat but throughout daily endeavors. This practice of constant mindfulness is taught universally by the yogis of the Himalayas, irrespective of their affiliations. There is no doubt, therefore, that smriti in this sutra is not ordinary memory, remembrance or recollection, but rather the practice of remaining intent upon self-observation, such as being mindful of breathing." [77]

samadhi

Though we have made considerable use of this term thus far in our study, this is its first appearance within the actual text of the yoga sutras. Samadhi is a state of mind which results when the mind is intensely absorbed as in meditation or prayer.

Samadhi is available to everyone. The ancient teachings tell us that even a mind that is normally distracted, even a disturbed mind, can settle into a state of samadhi.

But the samadhi of one mind may not be the equivalent of the samadhi of another in terms of clarity, discernment, steadiness, and the relative truth-bearing nature of the wisdom which results. There are many potential levels of samadhi which can manifest even within one individual mind.

prajna

Prajna is wisdom. The meaning here is the wisdom which arises through samadhi. The quality of prajna is dependent upon the quality and level of samadhi attained.

At the highest level, prajna demonstrates as the discernment of purusa. This discernment, when stabilized, leads in turn to paravairagya (transcendent dispassion) and ultimately to asamprajnata (a-cognitive) samadhi.

Ian Whicher speaks of the relation between prajna and pramana:

                                    Sutra - 20

"Ordinary valid cognition as understood in the Yoga-Sutra is...a sort of knowing wholly different from yogic "insight" (prajna). In its conventional usage, valid cognition is knowledge about reality (purusa and prakriti). Insight (prajna) is direct yogic perception ...and it purpose is to disclose knowledge of purusa. It may be concluded therefore that ordinary perception, inference, and valid testimony (authority) can produce correct knowledge about reality. But in Patanjali's system the above means of knowing (pramana) are merely instruments of conventional understanding, rational knowing, or even metaphysical knowledge, all of which can function as a buffer separating one from insight-by-direct-experience. Ordinary valid cognition is a mediated knowledge of purusa and prakriti; yogic insight or prajna... is immediate." [78]

purvaka

Purvaka, meaning preceded by, tells us that the necessary precondition for successful practice are the five factors enumerated here: faith, strength, mindfulness, samadhi, and samadhi-wisdom.

itaresam

Itaresam, of the others, refers back to sutras 1.18 and 1.19, pointing out the distinction between those who practice virama pratyaya, bhava pratyaya and upaya pratyaya.

Comments of a Contemporary Teacher

"This sutra suggests that faith, or confidence, gives us the energy, vitality, or even enthusiasm we need to overcome whatever distractions, doubts, or other obstacles arise, and enables us to remember where we are going. The combination of faith, energy, and strong memory enables us to override our past conditioning, and reorient our lives towards the highest Truth, or towards God, and sustain that orientation until the light of wisdom is achieved."

- Gary Kraftsow, American Viniyoga Institute [79]

—— Exploration ——

Amongst the "skillful means" presented here, a causal link is said to lead progressively from first to last. This suggests that conviction may manifest before one has developed the inner strength or the mindfulness with which to pursue a particular course, and that it is the wisdom gained from samadhi that may ultimately provide the necessary conditions for a-cognitive samadhi.

Conviction is a deep faith that there is some core truth in which we may safely place our trust and confidence. Implied is the belief that this core truth can be contacted and is personally available to each one of us. Faith comes about through a recognition that there is some power greater than the power of the individual mind.

Faith and conviction do not imply an abrogation of the mind. Discernment is just as necessary in the development and application of faith as it is in any other arena. Misplaced faith may

Sutra - 20

wreak great havoc for an individual or a community, and faith that is not balanced with wisdom may easily turn into fanaticism.

Inner strength comes from the conviction that there is some path worth trodding, and that one actually has the energy and persistence to trod it. Inner strength is what enables us to learn from our mistakes, to overcome our conditioning, to transmute weaknesses into virtues. Inner strength is the power to both temper the momentum and overcome the inertia of our daily lives.

Mindfulness is an active condition of undivided attention and presence of mind which reflects the unrelenting remembrance of the goal, the path and the means.

Samadhi, specifically cognitive samadhi, can manifest spontaneously even at its higher levels for many individuals. But such spontaneous occurrences regardless of their cause, whether they are due to grace or due to the merit of previous accomplishments, will not likely be maintained or stabilized without the developed trio of conviction, inner strength, and mindfulness.

As for wisdom, the kind of wisdom that is deep and lasting cannot be purchased by any means except the currency of authentic personal experience culled from real life situations which call forth the required resources.

———— **Further Reflections** ————

In the yoga sutra commentarial tradition there has been a recognition that in using the term itaresam, Patanjali is contrasting bhava pratyaya with the traditional practice of upaya pratyaya (though Patanjali does not utilize the term upaya here).

Interestingly, however, there has been a general failure to adequately recognize the juxtaposition of virama pratyaya with bhava pratyaya and upaya pratyaya.

Rather it is suggested that after Patanjali introduces virama pratyaya in 1.18, followed by the alternative path of bhava pratyaya in 1.19, he then backtracks in 1.20 to refer back to virama pratyaya, as if the application of skillful means are required for success in virama pratyaya, with upaya pratyaya being that means.

But Patanjali clearly states that a-cognitive samadhi preceded by virama pratyaya has only that impression which remains active as a remainder (a point on which there seems to be unanimous agreement).

This precludes the notion that a straight virama pratyaya practice requires other means applied for success, for then the residue of these other means would remain as active impressions and the practice would be rightfully referred to as one of skillful means or upaya pratyaya.

The fact that virama pratyaya is a path in and of itself is an important point, not just some intellectual roundabout.

First of all, it is important because there are some practitioners who are best suited to the direct path that virama pratyaya provides. Secondly, by reducing the number of possible paths presented to two rather than three, the subtle introduction of the three possible paths of the yogi (that correlate with the three primary spiritual paths which form the basis of spiritual traditions across the globe) will likely be missed.

Chapter 1, Sutra 21
—— *Offering* ——

Now is a good time.
All attainments are only a succession of 'nows.'

- Margo Morris

1.21 tīvrasaṃvegānāmāsannaḥ

tīvrasaṃvegānāmāsạnnaḥ

Translations

tivra	-	1. strong, intense 2. acute, sharp 3. fierce, violent
from tu:	-	to make strong or efficient
samveganam	-	1. with vehemence, ardor 2. with speed, velocity, force 3. with desire for emancipation
from vega:	-	1. a stream, flood, current 2. impetus, momentum 3. speed, haste, quickness

(Continued)

```
asannah          -        1. near, close
                          2. imminent

from asad:        -        1. to sit, sit near
                          2. to lie in wait for
                          3. to approach, meet with,
                          reach
```

1.21 When intense (with) fervent momentum it is near.

—— Introductory Remarks ——

Our subject matter here is still the attainment of asamprajnata or a-cognitive samadhi.

tivra

Tivra and samveganam are often rendered by similar or nearly identical terms, resulting in translations that amount to something like "intense intensity".

Tivra has the connotation of the degree of force applied to a particular object and is akin to the degree of willful effort (yatna - see sutra 1.13) which one exerts in one's practice. As such, the only realistic measurement of tivra is that which reflects a long-term perspective.

samveganam

Samvega, on the other hand, has to do with momentum, and momentum has to do with motion in a particular direction. Samvega in this context is one's overall momentum in relation to the goal of citta vritti nirodha.

We might say that tivra is the force, the ongoing willful effort that one applies to one's fervent momentum or samvega. Together they imply a practice imbued with a sense of immediacy.

Swami Veda Bharati , in his commentary, writes:

..."the derivative meaning of the word samvega includes vehemence, speed, velocity, force, momentum, rate of progress. By implication it means a strong samskara from the past and a strong ichchha – desire and will – to make fast progress." [80]

According to Swami Hariharananda Aranya:

"The word samvega is a technical term in the science of Yoga. We find it in Buddhist literature also. It means not only detachment but also aptitude combined with a feeling of reverence in devotional practice and the resultant ardor to hasten forward. It is like gathering momentum as you proceed." [81]

asannah

Asanna refers to one's goal - that it is very near or imminent when tivra samveganam is applied to one's practice. (Note: asanna is not be confused with asana, the practice of physical postures in yoga.)

—— **Exploration** ——

An appropriate practice is one that always takes into consideration the disposition, the level of development, and both the immediate and long term goals of the practitioner.

Patanjali's exhortation that "when intense with fervent momentum it is near" applies to everyone at all levels of practice, but it is particularly important in the yogi's attempt to bridge the gap between samprajnata samadhi and asamprajnata samadhi.

The current sutra focuses on the qualities of intensity and fervent momentum as they impact the three basic pratyaya paths, pratyaya being the underlying motivational, ideational and structural support of any given practice. In laying out the three types of pratyaya, Patanjali has underlined the differences between those who are naturally drawn to one path or the other based on the totality of their characteristics.

In order to assure a practice that will succeed, the yogi must ask:

What will bring a sense of **immediacy** to my practice? What will give rise to a sense of urgency, and harness the strength and vitality of my will and purpose?

The answer to these questions very much depends upon the attributes of the individual.

—— **Further Exploration** ——

A greater understanding of the three types of pratyaya requires historical context. Hindu religious philosophy and scripture is built around three primary Gods: Shiva, Vishnu and Brahma. These three Hindu Gods are analogous to the trinitarian Godhead of Buddhism, Zoroastrianism and Daoism as well as the Christian trinity of Father, Son and Holy Spirit. The three-fold spiritual path also presents in the Western Esoteric tradition as the Three Primary Rays.

1st Aspect of God, Shiva the Destroyer, the Father
2nd Aspect of God, Vishnu the Preserver, the Son
3rd Aspect of God, Brahma the Creator, the Holy Ghost

It is said that every individual's path is governed primarily by one of these three emanations of the Godhead. In the yoga sutras, the three basic streams (though not addressed in this manner) have not only provided a framework for ideational content, but have dictated the organization and presentation of its structural components.

If we look ahead to the upcoming sutras in Chapter 1, there is a general agreement that sutras 23-29 are descriptive of an alternative path. The implication, of course, is that one means has already been described (sutras 12-18), to which this second means is an alternative. Then along come sutras 30-39 which describe yet another path of overcoming obstacles through skillful means.

The overall structure of Chapter One may be analyzed as follows:

Sutras 1-11   -   Defines yoga in relation to the normal activities of the mind.

        -   Describes the five-fold nature of those activities and their potential positive and negative impact.

Sutras 12-17   -   Describes abhyasa and vairagya (practice and dispassion).

        -   Defines transcendent vairagya and introduces concept of purusa.

        -   Describes levels or grades of samprajnata (cognitive) samadhi.

        -   Points towards a-cognitive samadhi, transcending cognitive mind.

Sutras 18-22   -   Identifies virama pratyaya as a practice which precedes a-cognitive samadhi.

        -   Identifies bhava pratyaya as another practice leading to a-cognitive samadhi.

	-	Identifies practice of skillful means known as upaya pratyaya and enumerates five factors necessary for success.
	-	Describes relation of intensity and vehemence to success of practice
	-	Draws distinctions between mild, moderate and intense approach.

Sutras 23-29	-	Details the path of meditation on the Lord.
	-	Describes significance, use and purpose of the sacred syllable OM.
	-	Describes fruit of this path as the overcoming of all obstacles.

| Sutras 30-39 | - | Details the path of overcoming obstacles through the application of upaya pratyaya or skillful means. |

| Sutras 40-51 | - | Describes in detail the progressive states or levels of samadhi. |

Applying the three basic paths to the three types of pratyaya might render the following:

| virama pratyaya | - Intense pratyaya (seed-cognition of cessation - sutra 1.18) |

| bhava pratyaya | - Moderate pratyaya (seed-cognition of becoming - sutra 1.19) |

| upaya pratyaya | - Mild pratyaya (seed cognition of skillful means - sutra 1.20) |

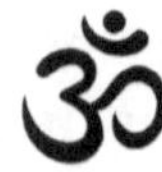

Chapter 1, Sutra 22
—— Offering ——

"Be soft in your practice, think of the method as a
fine silvery stream, not a raging waterfall.
Follow the stream, have faith in its course.
It will go on its way, meandering here, trickling there.
It will find the grooves, the cracks, the crevices.
Just follow it. Never let it out of your sight.
It will take you there."

- Buddhist Master Sheng-yen [82]

1.22 mṛdumadhyādhimātratvāt tato'pi viśeṣaḥ

mṛdu madhyādhimātratvāttato'pi viśeṣaḥ

Translations

mrdu	-	gentle, mild, slight
madhya	-	intermediate, moderate
adhimatratvat	-	intense, strong, of large measure
tato'pi	-	(tataha + api) even in that
visesa	-	difference, distinction, the distinguishing characteristic

1.22 Even in that there are distinctions between gentle, moderate and strong.

—— Introductory Remarks ——

Sutra 1.21 stated that when a practice is approached with intensity and fervent momentum, success is near. This applies regardless of the structure of the practice or the particular path chosen, though the path itself may be referred to as intense, moderate or mild.

In this study it is posited that there are three basic dispositions or temperaments of yogis, as follows:

1. Those of mild temperament whose aptitudes and traits lead them to a practice of upaya pratyaya resting on the meditative support of skillful means.

2. Those of moderate temperament who gravitate to a practice of bhava pratyaya resting on the meditative support of being or becoming.

3. Those of intense temperament who follow a practice of virama pratyaya and the meditative support of cessation.

Patanjali tells us that even within the overall framework of mild, moderate and intense, there are distinctions between gentle, moderate and strong application.

mrdu

Mrdu means gentle or mild.

madhya

Madhya connotes an intermediate or moderate level.

adhimatratvat

Adhimatratvat means intense or strong.

tato'pi

A contraction of tataha and api, tato'pi means due to that;
here: even in that.

visesa

Visesa is that which distinguishes one thing from another;
here: distinctions.

An Illustrative Story

*"We're familiar with going about errands in our car.
Usually, we allow for the expected obstructions and
delays. Traffic is heavy and slows us; we hit all the
stoplights, and perhaps there are accidents or even
an unreasonable policeman who scolds or gives us a
ticket. The air is heavy with exhaust fumes and the
noise of vehicles and horns jangle in our ears. Nearing
the destination, we find ourselves driving around the
block or many blocks in search of a parking place. We
arrive, at last, with nerves on edge, temper frayed, and
energy drained. A commonplace experience."*

*"Rarely, something quite different happens. We leave
the driveway and it seems as if everything is designed
to speed us on our way in the most carefree fashion.
Traffic flows; we only encounter green traffic lights.*

(Continued)

Without deviation we arrive at the shop we want and miraculously there is a parking place waiting for us right out front. (I assure the reader that such an occurrence is indeed a miracle in Chennai!) We can't escape the feeling that we must be doing exactly the right thing, at the right time, in the right place – even that there are invisible hands helping us along the way. A most un-commonplace experience!"

"And yet what is the real difference? The second trip that I have described was, of course, somewhat easier, somewhat quicker – all the external conditions seemed to favor us. The reality is despite the external conditions we achieved what we intended, what was necessary. That the usual journey was more difficult really makes little difference in the outcome"…"There is no reason why our first journey to the shop should not have left us feeling just as clear-minded, good-tempered, and energetic as the second."

- excerpt from T.K.V. Desikachar,
"Health, Healing and Beyond" [83]

Each of the three types of disposition listed above may be subdivided according to the intensity and the fervent momentum of the approach:

Mild pratyaya with gentle habitual application
Mild pratyaya with moderate habitual application
Mild pratyaya with strong habitual application

Moderate pratyaya with gentle habitual application
Moderate pratyaya with moderate habitual application
Moderate pratyaya with strong habitual application

Intense pratyaya with gentle habitual application
Intense pratyaya with moderate habitual application
Intense pratyaya with strong habitual application

Perhaps the point being made here is that one's natural temperament and disposition is not the sole factor determining one's approach to spiritual practice. Equally important is the level of intensity and momentum which the practitioner chooses to bring to the application of that practice.

——— **Further Reflections** ———

The path that leads to authentic fulfillment of our potential is none other than the unique path formed by our own process of self-discovery. What this means is for each of us to discover. In the course of our discovery we will make mistakes and misjudgments. Fortunately, through our mistakes we learn discernment.

By paying close attention, acknowledging cause and effect and making any necessary adjustments with patience and trust, we may come to be guided by a sensed inner truth, a knowingness that provides an ever-replenishing reserve of strength and energy. And slowly, sometimes painfully, we learn that the most profound truth of who we are as humans is not personal.

What name may we give to this sensed inner truth that serves as our guiding light, that steers us ever onward toward the actualization of our highest potential?

In naming it, we risk imprisonment by our own limited concepts. On the other hand, by naming it, we courageously expose our limited concepts to the purifying fires of our own introspection and the reflections we receive from others.

Whether we chose to name God or Lord, Christ or Isvara, purusa or Self, whether we seek Enlightenment or mystical union with the Divine, the words matter not. They all point to the same truth and the same place, that place which the ancient seers who transmitted these teachings called yoga.

Chapter 1, Sutra 23
—— Offering ——

Surrender ego and gain the world
Beyond my self, the Self unfurled
Seeing the Divine in all
Beyond the dogma, beyond the wall...

- Marc O'Maolain, from Ishvara Pranidhanam [84]

1.23 īśvarapraṇidhānādvā

īśvarapraṇidhānādvā

Translations

isvara (here: the Lord)	-	1. master, lord 2. the Supreme Being
pranidhanat	-	1. fixing, applying to, attention to 2. access, entrance 3. prayer, vow 4. profound religious meditation
va	-	or

1.23 Or by meditation on the Lord

—— Introductory Remarks ——

This sutra describes in detail the path of isvara pranidhana, meditation on the Lord.

isvara

Isvara is usually translated as Lord or Supreme Lord. The connotation varies slightly depending on the school of thought. In yoga traditions, the general implication of isvara is not that of a Creator God outside the world of form, but an emanation of God intimately involved with, yet separate from, the manifest world of form.

In Buddhism, isvara appears as Avalokiteshwara, the Lord as Witness, Bodhisattva of Compassion, who sits in meditation observing the world, remaining focused on the world as a service to others.

pranidhana

Pranidhana means to fix one's attention unwaveringly upon an object as in meditation or prayer. The traditional usage connotes a profound and continuous religious meditation, well-described by the phrase "practicing the presence of God".

va

Va (or) indicates an alternative to what has been presented.

—— Exploration ——

How does isvara relate to the Trimurti or the Trinity of God?

In Hindu scripture it is said that Shiva, Vishnu and Brahma are three aspects of isvara - that isvara is both Atman saguna (with form) as manifest in prakriti, as well as Atman nirguna (without form). Isvara is thus an umbrella term that encompasses all three aspects of God as God Incarnate.

The path of isvara pranidhana, being a path of devotion, is correlated with the second aspect of God. The predominant characteristic of the second aspect is devotional faith, the characteristic that binds us inexorably to the object of our devotion.

Vishnu - the second aspect of the Hindu Trimurti
Son of God - the second aspect of the Christian Trinity
Second Ray - the second aspect in Western Esoteric tradition

The idea in isvara pranidhana is to place full attention on the Highest, to wholeheartedly and faithfully dedicate our love and devotion to the Highest, knowing that in time, we ourselves will begin to reflect the Highest.

Sister Eileen O'Hea , who participated in a Christian Buddhist Seminar with H.H. the Dalai Lama which was chronicled in "The Good Heart, A Buddhist Perspective on the Teachings of Jesus" spoke thus:

"The Christian teaching has always been that we are made in God's image, that we are temples of the Holy Spirit, and that we are already in union with God. But because of our human condition, we don't experience it fully because we are still caught in our minds and our patterns. That is why we meditate and follow our spiritual practice so that we can return to what in Zen Buddhism is called our "original face", to that original experience of who we were created to be.... this does not involve a loss of identity, but is the experience of oneness with God". [87]

There is a similar theme in comments from Jean-Marie Dechenet in "Christian Yoga":

"The origin and cause of thoughts lies in the splitting up, by man's transgression, of his single and simple memory, which has thus lost the memory of God, and becoming multiple instead of simple, and varied instead of single, has fallen a prey to its own forces....To cure this original memory of the deceitful and harmful memory of thoughts means to bring it back to its ancient simplicity...Memory can be cured by a constant remembrance of God, consolidated by the action of prayer." [88]

—— **Further Reflections** ——

As discussed briefly in sutra 1.19 in relation to the path of the videhas and prakritilayas, when one is choosing to merge one's consciousness in religious meditation, when one is choosing to "become" the object of one's devotion, it is important to carefully choose that object with an eye to the ultimate results. Hence, Patanjali points to isvara.

A successful practice requiring deep faith must exist within a framework that the practitioner can commit to wholeheartedly.

In the words of H.H. the Dalai Lama:

"The belief in creation and divinity is not universal to all major religious traditions. While there are many traditions that base their practice and belief on that central premise, there are also certain traditions that do not. However, what is common to all religions is the importance of a firm grounding of one's spiritual practice on a single-pointed faith, or confidence, in an object of refuge...."

"In order to have such a single-pointed confidence and a sense of entrusting your spiritual well-being, one needs to develop a feeling of closeness and connectedness with those objects of faith." [89]

A successful practice must, of course, also be grounded in both reason and understanding.

Christina Feldman & Jack Kornfield, in "Stories of the Spirit, Stories of the Heart" wrote eloquently on the matter:

"Faith is a powerful double-edged sword. It has the potential to open our eyes or to blind us. Through wise faith we can surmount the greatest obstacle; through foolish faith we sentence ourselves to blind obedience. Faith can bring greater tolerance and humility or narrowness and bigotry. Faith can convince us that we are the custodians of truth; it can also open us to continue to learn from the challenges and mysteries of life."

"Wise faith opens rather than narrowing us. It encourages us to question, to explore, to inquire. It encourages us to discover our own answers and to trust in our own experience. Wise faith enables us to listen to and learn from the guidance and experience of others without being distracted from a deep inner trust that the power of transformation lies within us. The greatest faith is the faith that we have in ourselves to live as fully compassionate and loving human beings." [90]

Chapter 1, Sutra 24
—— *Offering* ——

God became man so that man might become God.

- Athanasius of Alexandria [91]

1.24 kleśakarmavipākāśayairaparāmṛṣṭaḥ
puruṣaviśeṣa īśvaraḥ

kle_śak_armavi_p_āk_āś_ayair_ap_ar_āmṛṣṭaḥ puruṣaviśeṣa īśv_araḥ

Translations

klesa	-	1. pain, affliction, distress 2. the five causes of suffering
karma (here: previous actions)	-	1. actions 2. field of action tied to beneficial or harmful results
vipaka	-	1. ripening, maturing (esp. the fruit of actions) 2. any change of form or state 3. effect, result, consequence

(Continued)

asaya	-	1. a receptacle or recipient
(here: latent		2. the 'stock' or balance of
impressions)		previous actions
apara-mrsta	-	untouched
purusa	-	the Spiritual Self (see 1.3 and 1.16)
visesa	-	distinctive, special
isvara	-	the Lord

1.24 Isvara is a special purusa untouched by the root causes of suffering, the consequences of previous actions, and latent impressions.

—— Introductory Remarks ——

Patanjali introduces the qualities of isvara.

klesa

Klesa refers to the five root causes of suffering, as noted in the discussion of sutra 1.5. They are:

1. avidya (ignorance of truth)
2. asmita (egoism, I-am-ness)
3. raga (attachment)
4. dvesa (aversion)
5. abhinivesa (longing for immortality).

karma

Karma is the relationship between actions and their consequences. It refers to the entire field of past actions, and is not limited to a particular incarnation.

Wasui Tatsuguchi, in "A Study of Shin Buddhism", writes on how karma functions in our lives:

"Despite the many predetermined forces acting upon the individual, we cannot dismiss the fact that there are also alternatives within a situation from which the individual may choose and act accordingly. It is true that we cannot exercise control over karma itself and therefore, we must accept what alternatives the situation affords us, as influenced by perpetual change. In this sense, karma as a principle of cause-and-effect determines much of what we are to do... karma itself is a neutral but active principle and according to how one sees it, it may be made to operate negatively or positively, [for] spontaneity and initiative are a part of the karmic process."

"The difference which makes karma function creatively and spontaneously lies within this confine of given alternatives. It is the basis of initiative with which we take on the given that makes the difference. We said that no one chooses the situation into which he is born, nor the equipment with which he is endowed when he comes into being as a individual personality. On the one hand, karma exercises a tremendous influence over us; but on the other, the way in which we apply ourselves in making the most out of life makes the difference whether living becomes meaningful or meaningless. This crucial matter of making the right choices within the light of the best known facts, decides whether we act rationally or irrationally." [92]

vipaka

Vipaka is the ripening or maturing of results and consequences, in this case, the consequences of previous actions.

asaya

Asaya refers to the subtlest latent impressions of past experiences. The implication here is that isvara is free of any latent impressions.

aparamrsta

Aparamrsta means untouched, unaffected.

purusa

As we saw in sutra 1.16, purusa is the unchanging pure consciousness which imbues life in human form and whose reality is not dependent upon material existence.

visesa

Visesa means distinctive or special. What is the meaning of "special purusa"?

An examination of this question usually starts with whether purusa is a singularity or plurality, i.e. whether or not each individual has a personal purusa or whether there is only one purusa, not many. Instead of taking on the singular vs. plural issue, it might be more useful to consider the matter from a somewhat different angle.

Rather than thinking of individuals, which invites dualistic questions, if we think of spiritual development as a progression of states of consciousness existing on successive stratum or levels, then whatever consciousness exists in one particular state or stratum simply resides there as part of that.

In that context, when we speak of purusa with distinctive characteristics, we are referring to a particular state of consciousness that exists at a particular level, with "special" in this case implying "of the highest order".

As to whether or not isvara was ever immersed in prakriti and subject to its characteristics, Patanjali states only that isvara is a special purusa unaffected by klesa, karma, vipaka and asaya.

isvara

Isvara is translated here as "the Lord".

Words Of A Master Poet

*In the ancient days, as the first quiver of speech graced my lips,
I ascended the holy mountain and spoke
unto God, saying "Master, I am thy slave.
Thy hidden will is my law and I shall obey thee forever more."*

But God made no answer, and departed like a mighty tempest.

*And after a thousand years I again ascended the holy mountain
and spoke unto God, saying, "Creator, I am thy creation.
Out of clay thou hast fashioned me and to thee I owe mine all."*

But God made no answer, and departed like a thousand swift wings.

*And after a thousand years I climbed the holy mountain
and spoke unto God again, saying, "Father, I am thy son.
In pity and love thou hast given me birth,
and through love and worship I shall inherit thy kingdom."*

*But God made no answer, and departed like the mist
that veils the distant hills.*

(Continued)

And after a thousand years I climbed the sacred mountain
and again spoke unto God, saying,
"My God, thou art my aim and my fulfillment;
I am thy yesterday and thou art my tomorrow.
I am thy root in the earth and thou art my flower in the sky,
and together we grow before the face of the sun."

Then God leaned over me, and in my ears
whispered words of sweetness,
and even as the stream that runs to the sea
is enfolded by her, he enfolded me.

- Kahlil Gibran, extract from "God" [93]

—————— **Exploration** ——————

When one is intentionally merging with an object of meditation in a devotional practice, the importance of carefully choosing the object of meditation cannot be overestimated. A devotional meditation at the highest level is what might be called an "identification" meditation, wherein the practitioner 'becomes" the object of devotion. By choosing isvara as the focus, the practitioner sets the course for purusa khyati, the realization of the true Self at the core of being.

Embedded in ancient tradition are meditation practices where the objects of meditation are gods, demigods and nature spirits. While there may be great value in such meditations, from an ultimate perspective a more direct path is to place one's heart and mind in the hands of the most all-encompassing emanation of God.

The following excerpt is from the teachings of Bhaktivedanta Swami Prabhupada:

"If the mystic yogî is diverted by the accompanying feats of mystic control, then his mission of yogic success is a failure, because the ultimate aim is God realization. He is therefore recommended to fix his gross materialistic mind by a different conception and thus realize the potency of the Lord. As soon as the potencies are understood to be instrumental manifestations of the transcendence, one automatically advances to the next step, and gradually the stage of full realization becomes possible for him."[94]

—— **Further Explorations** ——

From Swami Krishnananda's "The Philosophy of Life, Part One: The Foundations of Philosophy":

"God is not, strictly speaking, any arbitrary creator of the world but the primary principle responsible and necessary for the expression of an environment fitted to the manner in which the Karmas of the individuals have to fructify themselves in various ways..."

"The Lord speaks in the Bhagavad Gita: "I am the Vedic rite, I am the sacrifice, I am the food offered to the manas, I am the herbs and the medicines, I am the sacred formula and the hymn; I am the clarified butter (offered in sacrifices); I am the consecrated fire, I the oblation. I am the Father of this world, the Mother, Supporter, the Grandfather; I am the object to be known, I the purifier (of all things), the syllable OM, and also the sacred lore of the Rik, the Sama and the Yajus; the Goal, the Sustainer, the Lord, the Witness, the Abode, the Refuge, the Friend, the Origin, the Dissolution, the Basis, the Storehouse, the Imperishable Seed. I give heat, I send forth rain, and also withhold it; I am immortality and also death; I am being and also non-being, O Arjuna!"... [95]

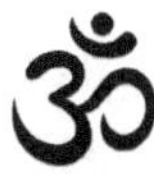

Chapter 1, Sutra 25
—— *Offering* ——

Because of Omniscience 'you are never alone'...
He knew of your end even before you were born.
And He's readied your mansion and has it adorned.

- Robert Edgar Burns, extract from "Omniscient" [96]

1.25 tatra niratiśayaṃ sarvajñabījam

tatra niratiśayaṃ sarvajñabījam

Translations

tatra (here: in Him)	-	there, in that place
niratisayam	-	unsurpassed, preeminent
from atisaya:	-	preeminence, superiority
sarvajna	-	omniscient, the all-knowing
from sarva:	-	all, every, entire
+ jna:	-	to know
bijam	-	1. primary cause or principle 2. source, origin 3. seed

1.25 In Him (the) preeminent seed of all-knowingness.

—— Introductory Remarks ——

tatra

Tatra means "in Him" or in that place, referring here to isvara.

niratisayam

Nitarasyam means preeminent. As a special purusa, unaffected by klesa, karma, vipaka and asaya, isvara is preeminent.

sarvajna

Sarvajna means omniscient, all-knowing.

bijam

Bijam is the seed, the origin of consciousness, the cause of all-knowingness.

A Christian Perspective

"There is...an attitude..it may be called threskeia in Greek, but in Latin religio, the religion which "binds" us to God...which in default of one equivalent word we may call 'worship' of God. What is expressed by those words is the worship we hold to be due only to Him who is the true God, who transforms his worshipers into gods."

- Saint Augustine, City of God [97]

The ultimate purpose of practice is the realization of purusa, the realization of the Self.

As mentioned in the discussion of sutra 1.19, there are differences between Buddhist and Hindu traditions when it comes to the notion of an individualized purusa.

While some teachings of Hinduism and Samkhya posit the existence of an individualized Self or "personal" purusa, Buddhism emphatically refutes that an individualized self could ever be considered an ultimate ground of reality. In Buddhism isvara appears as Avalokitesvara and Mahaisvara. Both are considered to be great Bodhisattvas who have attained liberation yet remain connected to the worldly realms in order to help others in their quest for liberation.

For some, it be may advisable, once again, to temporarily side-step this issue of whether purusa is a singularity or a plurality. That may be the most practical approach for the practitioner. After all, as yogis we always strive to remain open to making adjustments in our practice as needed.

In the relative sense, what matters is the state of consciousness we manage to bring to our practice. And in the ultimate sense, what matters is the state of consciousness we manage to bring to our lives. It is not the words or the names that define the results of our efforts, it is the attributes which we embrace.

—— **Further Reflections** ——

As with every element which we choose for our personal practice, there should be an authentic inner resonance that allows for an ever-deepening understanding and experience of the true nature of our being. What brings on such an authentic resonance will depend upon many factors. Thus, we must be ever-attentive and ever-vigilant in our choices.

For "it is better to live your own destiny imperfectly than to live an imitation of somebody else's life with perfection."

As spoken by Lord Krishna in the Bhagavad Gita:

"The soul is neither born, nor does it ever die; nor having once existed, does it ever cease to be. The soul is without birth, eternal, immortal, and ageless. It is not destroyed when the body is destroyed."...

"The power of God is with you at all times; through the activities of mind, senses, breathing, and emotions; and is constantly doing all the work using you as a mere instrument."

Chapter 1, Sutra 26
—— Offering ——

For the love of God is broader
Than the measure of man's mind....

- F. Faber, from "There's a Wideness in God's Mercy" [98]

1.26 sa eṣa pūrveṣāmapi guruḥ
kālenānavacchedāt

sa eṣa pūrveṣāmapi guruḥ kālenānavacchedāt

Translations

sa esa	-	this very one
purvesam	-	1. antecedent, earlier 2. of the ancients, the first
api	-	even
guru	-	spiritual teacher or preceptor
kalena	-	in time, over a long time from: kala (time)
anavacchedat	-	1. undivided, uncut 2. uncurtailed, unbounded

(Continued)

> from avacchedat: - 1. anything cut off, separated
> 2. distinctive, particularized

1.26 This very one, unbounded by time, is the teacher of even the ancient teachers.

—— Introductory Remarks ——

sa esa

Sa esa means this very one.

purvesam

The meaning of purvesam is antecedent. Here it refers to isvara, indicating that isvara is the antecedent teacher, the first teacher.

api

Api means even.

guru

According to the Advayataraka Upanishad, gu means darkness and ru means that which dispels darkness.

As an adjective guru means heavy, "with gravitas". Guru connotes a spiritual teacher or guide, signifying one who not only imparts knowledge, but leads the way and unveils the path for the spiritual aspirant.

Reverend Jaganath Carrera, founder of Yoga Life Society, on the subject of gurus:

"It is important to realize the central place the Guru holds in Indian thought, and in all mystic traditions, East and West. The Guru is not what many today imagine. The Guru is not just a master teacher or speaker. Some Gurus spoke little or not at all. The Guru is not just the intelligence of an individual or the knowledge accumulated from years of study. The Guru is a conduit or embodiment of the qualities of Isvara...historically, great enlightened individuals were addressed as Isvara, a practice that continues to this day." [99]

kalena

Kala is time. Kalena means over the course of a long period of time, throughout time.

anavacchedat

Anavacchedat means uncut, unbounded, referring to kalena. The suggestion is that isvara is unchanging and unbounded throughout time and remains untouched by the cycle of samsara.

An Historical Perspective

"In the yogic lore, Shiva is seen as the first yogi or Adiyogi, and the first Guru or Adi Guru. Several Thousand years ago, on the banks of the lake Kantisarovar in the Himalayas, Adiyogi poured his profound knowledge into the legendary Saptarishis or "seven sages". The sages carried this powerful yogic science to different parts of the world...."

- Dr. Ishwar V. Basavaraddi [100]

——— **Exploration** ———

In speaking of the teacher of even the first teachers, Patanjali is speaking historically, but the connotation is far more than just historical. It is metaphysical. The Divine spark that resides in each of us has a direct link to God. This means that within each of us there is a pure, pristine and unchanging awareness. This Self, unaffected by the sufferings or pleasures of existence in human form, is the part of isvara that resides within us, the eternal connection with God that is inherently ours.

The teacher of even the ancients has always been and will always be the same. That is our human destiny.

——— **Further Reflections** ———

Self realization is a place, a place we find within ourselves when we peel away the doubts, uncertainties and limitations that cloud our ability to know what is real. Isvara is a state of consciousness which we are invited to share.

Swami Sivananda in "JnanaYoga" states:

"When the Jiva sheds its cramping individuality, it finds itself in an experience of the majestic Unity of beings." [101]

Chapter 1, Sutra 27
—— *Offering* ——

Om is the sound of the Lord most worshipful.
We meditate on the Lord and his Glory.
May he illumine our hearts and our minds.

- Gyatri Mantra

In the beginning was the Word
and the Word was with God
and the Word was God.

- John 1:1, the Bible

1.27 tasya vācakaḥ praṇavaḥ

tasya vācakaḥ praṇavaḥ

Translations

tasya	-	Him
from ta:	-	that one
+ sya:	-	3rd person pronoun
(Continued)		

---

vacakah	-	1. speaking, saying, declaring 2. expressive of, signifying 3. verbal, expressed by words 4. a messenger
pranavah	-	1. fore-sound, primeval sound 2. the mystical or sacred symbol Om
from pranu:	-	1. to roar, bellow, sound, reverberate 2. to utter the syllable Om

1.27 Om is the word which expresses Him.

—— Introductory Remarks ——

Patanjali states that Om is the word, the name, the sound that expresses isvara.

tasya

Tasya is a third person pronoun (him, her, it) referring here to isvara.

vacaka

The root of vacaka is vac, which means speech, language, or sound.

pranava

Pranava refers to the sacred syllable Om. It is the sound, the essence, of isvara.

From The Bhagavad Gita

"With your whole heart surrender to the divine presence at the core of your being, and by the grace of that divine presence, experience the silence of its timeless abode."

—— Exploration ——

Sacred scriptures tell us that Om is the primordial sound from which the world was created.

The use of the Om (AUM) dates back at least 5000 years to the scriptures of the Vedic period, where it was regarded as the most sacred of all mantras. The yoga sutras teach that Om is the bija, or seed mantra, of all other mantras.

In Devanagari, the system of phonetic symbols for writing Sanskrit, the symbol of Om is a cursive ligature comprised of the letters A, U and M.

The proper pronunciation of Om is tri-syllabic A-U-M. (Om is a transliteration...O being a diphthong of A + M).

Each letter of AUM corresponds to a state of consciousness:

A - waking state
U - dream state
M - deep sleep state

In the Devanagari symbol, above the A-U-M ligature, there is an upward curved line representing maya, the illusion of everyday existence. Above that curved line is a singular dot representing turiya, the "fourth state" – freedom.

The silence at the end of an AUM invocation is said to contain this fourth state, turiya, which is beyond space and time.

The three syllables A-U-M are also said to represent the trimurti or the three aspects of God (Shiva, Vishnu and Brahma) as well as the three gunas (rajas, sattva and tamas).

Edwin Bryant, in his commentary on the sutras, wrote the following:

> "The mantra pranava, or AUM, is both the sound symbol of Isvara and the means for realization of Isvara. With repetition of AUM, the meaning of Isvara is understood. The relationship between Isvara and AUM is not just a designation or a name based on language. Rather, it is inherent in the relationship between the word and the meaning. Pranava, AUM, is the word and Isvara is the meaning. The connection is eternal and inseparable. One does not exist without the other. Ultimately, Isvara is not the object of the search; it is the subject of the search. The end result is the realization that Isvara is within. And when we grasp this, we realize that purusha, our own true Self, and Isvara are one." [102]

Nischala Joy Devi, in "The Secret Power of Yoga, A Woman's Guide to the Heart and Spirit of the Yoga Sutras" wrote:

> "When expressed with great devotion, the sacred sound reveals our Divine Nature. The sacred sound must pluck the strings of our heart in order to unite our entire being with our true Divine Nature." [103]

"I am That I am" is a statement found in the Bible, in the Book of Exodus. It is the response that God gave to Moses when Moses asked God for his name. The phrase is generally understood to mean that God is self-existent and eternal, and that he needs no explanation for his being.

Ramana Maharshi, the great Indian sage declared that of all the definitions of God, "none is indeed so well put as the biblical statement 'I am That I am'".

Hebrew speakers generally note that the translation of "I am That I am" into English loses the subtleties of the original Hebrew text, which simultaneously connotes past, present and future, while also suggesting a sense of "I am with you even now."

In Christianity, theologians point to the difference between Christ and Jesus. Christ is the Spiritual name of Jesus, the name Jesus obtained upon the realization of his Christhood.

This dual nature of Jesus and Christ exemplifies the difference between the "I am-ness" of asmita and the "I am That I am" of isvara.

There is great power in the invocation of a name. When invoking the sacred sound OM, the divine essence is called forth in the one uttering the sound.

Chapter 1, Sutra 28
—— Offering ——

Just by repeating the name,
That which can not be understood
Will be understood.
Just by repeating the name,
That which can not be seen Will be seen...

- Anonymous

1.28 tajjapastadarthabhāvanam

tajjapastadarthābhāvanam

Translations

taj (tat)	-	that
japa (here: recitation)	-	1. whispering, muttering 2. repeating prayers or names of a deity
from jap:	-	1. to utter in a low voice 2. to pray in a low voice 3. to invoke or call upon
tad (tat)	-	that

(Continued)

---

artha (here: meaning)	-	1. purpose or aim 2. what is intended or meant
bhavanam (here: being absorbed in)	-	1. to occupy one's thoughts with 2. to direct one's thoughts towards 3. to be engaged or engrossed in
from bhava:	-	being, becoming

1.28 Recitation of that (for) being absorbed in its meaning.

—— Introductory Remarks ——

tat

Tat refers to pranava, the sacred syllable OM, as introduced in 1.27.

japas

Japa refers to whispering or praying in a low voice, as in repetition of a syllable or name.

tadartha

Tadartha connotes meaning, referring here to the meaning of OM.

bhavanam

Bhavanam indicates being absorbed or engrossed in something. It is derived from bhava, meaning being or becoming.

——— **Exploration** ———

The phrase bhava pratyaya was introduced in sutra 1.19. In the discussion of that sutra, bhava pratyaya is translated as "seed cognition of becoming". This is the path of religious devotion, the path of the Lord, of "becoming God".

The repetition of Om is the means on this path. Through repetition, the invocation of Om becomes an established pattern within the being of the practitioner. The traditional methodology in the repetition of OM is to either employ a hushed voice or to perform the repetition silently.

When we invoke the word OM, the sacred sound of isvara, we are aligning ourselves mentally, emotionally and physiologically with that sacred energy. Through OM, we call the energy of isvara to ourselves and at the same time call forth that energy within ourselves.

It is akin to the creation of an electrical circuit with a continuous flow of current between two nodes. When the flow becomes well established, the practitioner is in a position to know that the two nodes of the circuit are, in essence, the same.

The Mundaka Upanishad describes Om as the bow, atma (the soul) as the arrow; and Brahman as the target:

> "Affix to the Upanishad, the bow incomparable, the sharp arrow of devotional worship; then, with mind absorbed and heart melted in love, draw the arrow and hit the mark– the imperishable Brahman. Om is the bow, the arrow is the individual being, and Brahman is the target. With a tranquil heart, take aim. Lose thyself in him, even as the arrow is lost in the target".

From the Svetasvatara Upanishad, on the meaning of Om:

"The servant requested of the King two pieces of fire wood and then asked 'can you please show me the fire inside this wood?' The King was unable to do so. The servant then placed the two pieces of firewood together and began to churn them. When a fire ignited the servant said 'O King, though it is not visible, the fire is already present inside the fire wood."

—— Further Reflections ——

In sutra 1.18 Patanjali stated that a-cognitive samadhi which is preceded only by the practice of virama pratyaya (the seed-cognition of cessation), has only that habitual potency as residue.

In the same way, we may infer that a-cognitive samadhi preceded only by the practice of bhava pratyaya (the seed-cognition of becoming), has only that habitual potency as residue. The key to a successful attenuation of habitual potency in the case of bhava pratyaya is the choice of what one is committing oneself to become.

When choosing isvara as the object of meditation and devotion, and when absorbing oneself in isvara through repetition of OM, the outcome of a-cognitive samadhi has only "becoming isvara" as the residue.

Chapter 1, Sutra 29
—— *Offering* ——

There is a life-force within your soul, seek that life.
There is a gem in the mountain of your body,
seek that mine.
O traveler, if you are in search of That
Don't look outside, look inside yourself and seek That.

- Jalal Al-din Rumi, extract from 'Thief of Sleep" [104]

1.29 tataḥ pratyakcetanādhigamo'pyantarāyābhāvaśca

tataḥ pratyakcetanādhigamo'pyantarāyābhāvaśca

Translations

tata	-	then
pratyak	-	1. turned inward
		2. turned back, averted
		3. backwards, in an opposite direction
cetana	-	1. of the citta
		2. that which comes from the citta
		3. consciousness, awareness
		4. intentions, volition

(Continued)

adhigama   -   1. the act of acquiring (knowledge)
(here: realization)   2. acquiring spiritual mastery
                       3. realization of truth

from adhi-gam: to go up to

api   -   as well as

antaraya   -   obstacles, hindrances

abhavasca   -   absence

1.29 Then the realization of the inward turned consciousness and the absence of obstacles.

—— Introductory Remarks ——

This completes the explanation of the path of isvara pranidhana.

tata

Tata means then.

pratyak

Pratyak means turned inward, back, in an opposite direction.

This brings us back to our discussion of sutra 1.2:

"Another useful image comes from the second meaning of rodha which, when combined with ni, suggests the image of a sprouting seed whose normal process of outward and upward growth is turned back toward some innate inner potential."

cetana

Cetana is derived from cit, sharing the same root as the word citta. The literal meaning is "of the citta" or that which comes from the citta.

Again, from the discussion of sutra 1.2:

"As the citta comes into contact with its objects of perception, it is affected by the interaction. This is the normal activity to which the perceiving mind is habituated. But behind this normal process lies a "supranormal" state of consciousness which remains "unmodified" by the mind or the activities of the mind."

Pratyak and cetana, taken together, literally means "an inward turning of that which comes from the citta," and points directly to citta vritti nirodha.

adhigama

Adhigama means "to go up to", as in two things coming nearer. It suggests a process of learning, of gaining a new knowledge or understanding. In the current context it further cements the idea that an equivalence is being drawn between pratyak cetana adhigama and citta vritti nirodha.

Adhigama is part of a contrasting word pair, with the other word being agama. Agama means 'to go down to' as opposed to adhigama 'to go up to'; one is descending and the other is ascending. Traditional knowledge, most especially scriptural knowledge, is referred to as agama.

In Buddhism, adhigama-dharma refers to personal realization, while agama-dharma, refers to the body of knowledge transmitted through the scriptures.

api

Api means "as well as".

antaraya

Antaraya refers to obstacles, impediments.

abhava

Abhava means absence.

ca

Ca is "and" or "also".

A Buddhist View

Agama and Adhigama are the Buddhist terms for descent and ascent, connoting salvation from above and self-realization from below:

"Ascent can be understood as an activity or movement from this world to the world yonder, or from this human personal existence to the impersonal...these two activities function in opposite directions, so they tend to be paradoxical, at times illogical, even contradictory. But, in fact, it is this "two-directional activity"... that constitutes the characteristic feature of the Mahayana. [105]

- Gadjin M. Nagao, Presidential Address, Intl Association of Buddhist Studies

—— Exploration ——

It is clear that an understanding of these ancient truths is not limited to particular societies or geographical regions. The following words are from the ancient Gnostic scripture, the Corpus Hermeticum:

"The path back to your Divine Father leads beyond your body, from which you must shift your attention. Your thoughts, feelings, and sensations arise from contact with matter; you must release them. Move upward through the seven spheres of your being into the highest region of your awareness. Let go of everything else and merge your awareness in God alone. Do this not for your own sake, but so that you can help others."

—— Further Reflections ——

The descent of grace and Realization of the Self are the same. A spiritual awakening is an uncovering of the innate potentialities of consciousness. It matters not whether we adhere to a prescribed path laid out before us or whether we navigate the uncharted waters through the compass of our own inner guidance. What matters is that we strive to bring the best of what we have to give. The rest is letting go. The rest takes care of itself.

Words From A Master Poet

Traveler, your footprints
are the only road, nothing else.
Traveler, there is no road;
you make your own path as you walk.
As you walk, you make your own road,
and when you look back
you see the path
you will never travel again.
Traveler, there is no road;
only a ship's wake in the sea.

- Antonio Machado, There Is No Road [107]

—— Endnotes ——

1 Swami Veda Bharati (Usharbudh Arya), Yoga Sutras of Patanjali (Honesdale, Pennsylvania: Himalayan International Institute, 1986)

2 T.K.V. Desikachar, Patanjali's Yogasutras (Madras: Affiliated East-West Press Private Limited, 1987)

3 Arthur Osborne, "Be Still" Poetry for the Spirit (London Watkins Publishing, 1999)

4 Tirumalai Krishnamacharya, Yoganjalisaram (Chennai, India: Krishnamacharya Yoga Mandiram, 1976)

5 H.H. the Dalai Lama, The Good Heart: A Buddhist Perspective On The Teachings Of Jesus (Boston: Wisdom Publications, 1996)

6 Jalal Al-din Rumi,"The Churn" (source unknown)

7 Sir Monier Monier-Williams, A Sanskrit-English Dictionary (Delhi: Motilal Banarsidass Publishers Private Limited, 1963)

8 H.H. the Dalai Lama, The Good Heart: A Buddhist Perspective On The Teachings Of Jesus (Boston: Wisdom Publications, 1996)

9 Jalal Al-din Rumi, "The Well" (source unknown)

10 Jalal Al-Din Rumi, "Masnavi" (source unknown)

11 T. K. V. Desikachar, Patanjali's Yogasutras (Madras, India: Affiliated East-West Press Private Ltd., 1987)

12   Stephen Pinker, How The Mind Works
(New York & London: W.W. Norton &Company, 1997)

13   Jalal Al-Din Rumi (source unknown)

14   H.H. The Dalai Lama, "Where Buddhism Meets
Neuroscience" (Boulder, CO: Shambhala Publications,
1999)

15   H.H. The Dalai Lama, Kindness, Clarity, and Insight
(Delhi: Motilal Banarsidass Publishers Private Limited,
1997)

16   Jalal Al-Din Rumi (source unknown)

17   T.K.V. Desikachar, Patanjali's Yogasutras (Madras:
Affiliated East-West Press Private Limited, 1987)

18   Sir Monier Monier-Williams, A Sanskrit-English
Dictionary (Delhi: Motilal Banarsidass Publishers
Private Limited, 1963)

19   Kabir Edmund Helminski, Living Presence (New York:
Jeremy P. Tarcher/G.P. Putnam's Sons, 1992)

20   H.D. "The Walls Do Not Fall" (New York, Liveright
Publishing, 1925)

21   Swami Hariharananda Aranya, Yoga Philosophy of
Patanjali (Albany, N.Y.: SUNY Press, 1983)

22   Christopher DeCharms, Two Views of Mind
(New York: Snow Lion Publications, 1998)

23   Michael C. Corballis, The Lopsided Ape
(New York/Oxford: Oxford University Press, 1991)

24.   Ibid.

25   The Dalai Lama, et al, Consciousness At The Crossroads
(Ithaca, N.Y.: Snow Lion Publications, 1999)

26   The Dalai Lama, et al, Sleeping, Dreaming and Dying
(Boston: Wisdom Publications, 1997)

27   Ibid.

28   Ibid.

29   Ibid.

30   Ibid.

31   The Dalai Lama, et al, Consciousness At The Crossroads
(Ithaca, N.Y.: Snow Lion Publications, 1999)

32   Ibid.

33   James McConkey, The Anatomy of Memory
(New York: Oxford University Press, 1996)

34   Ralph Waldo Emerson, Journals (October 27, 1831)

35   Hilts, Philip J., Memory's Ghost (New York: Touchstone,
1995)

36   James McConkey, The Anatomy of Memory
(New York: Oxford University Press, 1996)

37   Ibid.

38   A. R. Ammons, "Pet Panther", Lake Effect Country
(New York: W.W. Norton, 1983)

39   Bernard Bouanchaud, The Essence Of Yoga
        (Portland, Oregon: Rudra Press, 1997)

40   Ganganatha Jha, Yoga-Sara-Sangraha of Vijnana-
        Bhiksu (Delhi, India: Parimal Publications, 1995)

41   Swami Veda Bharati (Usharbudh Arya), Yoga Sutras of
        Patanjali (Honesdale, Pennsylvania: Himalayan
        International Institute, 1986)

42   V.S. Ramachandran, M.D. and Sandra Blakeslee,
        Phantoms In The Brain (New York: William Morrow
        and Company, Inc., 1998)

43   Ibid.

44   Ibid.

45   Ibid.

46   Jalal Al-din Rumi, "Open the Window" (source unknown)

47   Swami Veda Bharati (Usharbudh Arya), Yoga Sutras of
        Patanjali (Honesdale, Pennsylvania: Himalayan
        International Institute, 1986)

48   H. H. the Dalai Lama, The Art of Happiness (New York:
        Riverhead Books, Penguin Putnam Inc., 1998)

49   St. Augustine. City of God (first published 1467)
        (Harmondsworth, England: Penguin Books Ltd., 1984)

50   Swami Rama, Living With The Himalayan Masters
        (Honesdale, Pennsylvania; Himalayan Intl.Institute 1978)

51   Mechtild of Magdeburg (source unknown)

52   Swami Hariharananda Aranya, Yoga Philosophy of
      Patanjali (Albany,N.Y.: SUNY Press, l983)

53   Bangali Baba, Yogasutra of Patanjali (Delhi, India:
      Motilal Banarsidass, 1976)

54   Ganganatha Jha, Yoga-Sara-Sangraha of Vijnana-
      Bhiksu (Delhi, India: Parimal Publications, 1995)

55   Ramana Maharshi, The Spiritual Teaching of Ramana
      Maharshi (Tiruvanamalai, India: Sri Ramanasramam,
      1972)

56   Sir Monier Monier-Williams, A Sanskrit-English
      Dictionary (Delhi: Motilal Banarsidass Publishers
      Private Limited, 1963)

57   Vasant Lad, "Strands of Eternity" (Albuquerque, NM:
      Ayurvedic Press, 2004)

58   Swami Veda Bharati (Usharbudh Arya), Yoga Sutras of
      Patanjali (Honesdale, Pennsylvania: Himalayan
      International Institute, l986)

59   Georg Feuerstein, The Yoga-Sutra Of Patanjali (Roches-
      ter, Vermont: Inner Traditions International, 1979)

60   Swami Veda Bharati (Usharbudh Arya), Yoga Sutras of
      Patanjali (Honesdale, Pennsylvania: Himalayan
      International Institute, l986)

61   Swami Hariharananda Aranya, Yoga Philosophy Of
      Patanjali (Albany, New York: SUNY Press, 1983)

62   Swami Veda Bharati (Usharbudh Arya), Yoga Sutras of
      Patanjali (Honesdale, Pennsylvania: Himalayan
      International Institute, l986)

63   Trevor Leggett, The Chapter Of The Self (London and
      Henley: Routledge & Paul Kegan 1978)

64   John Clare, "I Am!" (source unknown)

65   Swami Veda Bharati (Usharbudh Arya), Yoga Sutras of
      Patanjali (Honesdale, Pennsylvania: Himalayan
      International Institute, 1986)

66   Jalal-Al-Din Rumi (source unknown)

67   Swami Veda Bharati (Usharbudh Arya), Yoga Sutras of
      Patanjali (Honesdale, Pennsylvania: Himalayan
      International Institute, 1986)

68   Fernando Tola, Carmen Dragonetti, The Yogasutras Of
      Patanjali [English translation by K. D. Prithipaul] (Delhi:
      Motilal Barasidass Publishers Pvt. Ltd., 1991)

69   Ian Whicher, The Integrity of the Yoga Darsana
      (New York: State University of New York Press, 1998)

70   William Blake, "The Lamb" (source unknown)

71   Tejo Bindu Upanishad

72   Geshe Kelsang Wangmo, The Four Schools of Buddhist
      Philosophy, Tushita Meditation Centre Course Materials

73   Sir Monier Monier-Williams, A Sanskrit-English
      Dictionary (Delhi: Motilal Banarsidass Publishers
      Private Limited, 1963)

74   Ian Whicher, The Integrity of the Yoga Darsana
      (New York: State University of New York Press, 1998)

75   Swami Hariharananda Aranya, Yoga Philosphy Of
      Patanjali (Albany, New York: SUNY Press, 1983)

76   Gary Kraftsow, American Viniyoga Institute, 1992

77   Swami Veda Bharati (Usharbudh Arya), Yoga Sutras of
      Patanjali (Honesdale, Pennsylvania: Himalayan
      International Institute, l986)

78   Ian Whicher, The Integrity of the Yoga Darsana
      (New York: State University of New York Press, 1998)

79   Gary Kraftsow, American Viniyoga Institute, 2024

80   Swami Veda Bharati (Usharbudh Arya), Yoga Sutras of
      Patanjali (Honesdale, Pennsylvania: Himalayan
      International Institute, l986)

81   Swami Hariharananda Aranya, Yoga Philosophy Of
      Patanjali (Albany, New York: SUNY Press, 1983)

82   Chan Master Sheng Yen, "Getting the Buddha Mind"
      (New York: Dharma Drum Publications, 1982)

83   T.K.V. Desikachar, The Heart of Yoga (Rochester, VT:
      Inner Traditions, 1999)

84   Marc O'Maolain, extract from "Ishvara Pranidhanam"
      (Philippines: online source - poemhunter.com)

85   Wasui Tatsuguchi, A Study of Shin Buddhism
      (Honolulu: Shinshu Kyokai Mission Of Hawaii, 1961)

86   Jean-Marie Dechenet, Christian Yoga
      (New York: Harper & Row Publishers, 1960)

87   H.H. the Dalai Lama, The Good Heart: A Buddhist
Perspective On The Teachings Of Jesus (Boston: Wisdom
Publications, 1996)

88   Jean-Marie Dechenet, Christian Yoga
(New York: Harper & Row Publishers, 1960)

89   H.H. the Dalai Lama, The Good Heart: A Buddhist
Perspective On The Teachings Of Jesus (Boston: Wisdom
Publications, 1996)

90   Christina Feldman & Jack Kornfield, Stories of the Spirit,
Stories of the Heart (New York: Harper Collins
Publishers, 1991)

91   Athanasius of Alexandria (source unknown)

92   Wasui Tatsuguchi, A Study of Shin Buddhism
(Honolulu: Shinshu Kyokai Mission Of Hawaii, 1961)

93   Kahlil Gibran (source unknown)

94   Swami Krishnananda "The Philosophy of Life, Part One:
The Foundations of Philosophy, Chapter 9: Isvara or the
Universal Soul (online source)

95   Ibid.

96   Robert Edgar Burns, Complete Poetical Works of
Robert Burns (New York: T. Y. Crowell & Co. 1884)

97   St. Augustine. City of God (first published 1467)
(Harmondsworth, England: Penguin Books Ltd., 1984)

98   Frederick W. Faber, "There's a Wideness in God's Mercy"
(source unknown)

99   Reverend Jaganath Carrera, founder of Yoga Life Society (online source)

100   Dr. Ishwar V. Basavaraddi, "Yoga: Its Origin, History and Development" (online source)

101   Bhaktivedanta Swami Prabhupada, "Srimad-Bhâgavatam" (Delhi: League of Devotees, Vrindaban, 1962)

102   Edwin F. Bryant, The Yoga Sutras of Patanjali (New York: Northpoint Press, 2013)

103   Nischala Joy Devi, The Secret Power of Yoga, A Woman's Guide to the Heart and Spirit of the Yoga Sutras (Louisville, KY: Harmony House 2022)

104   Jalal Al-Din Rumi (source unknown)

105   Gadjin M. Nagao,"Ascent and Descent: Two Direction-Activity in Buddhist Thought", (Presidential Address for The Sixth Conference of The IABS, Tokyo, Japan, Sept, 1983 - online source)

106   Pir Hazrat Inayat Khan, "The Teaching of Pir Hazrat Inayat Khan" (Vol. 4, Mental Purification, Section 3. "Unlearning" - online source)

107   Antonio Machado, There is no Road (source unknown)

—— Bibliography ——

Ammons, A.R., "Pet Panther", Lake Effect Country (New York: W.W. Norton, 1983)

Aranya, Swami Hariharananda, Yoga Philosophy of Patanjali (Albany, N.Y.: SUNY Press, 1983)

Athanasius of Alexandria (source unknown)

Augustine, St., City of God (first published 1467) (Harmondsworth, England: Penguin Books Ltd., 1984)

Bangali Baba, Yogasutra of Patanjali (Delhi, India: Motilal Banarsidass, 1976)

Basavaraddi, Dr. Ishwar V., "Yoga: Its Origin, History and Development" (online source)

Bharati, Swami Veda (Usharbudh Arya), Yoga Sutras of Patanjali (Honesdale, Pennsylvania: Himalayan International Institute, l986)

Blake, William, "The Lamb" (source unknown)

Bouanchaud, Bernard, The Essence Of Yoga (Portland, Oregon: Rudra Press, 1997)

Bryant, Edwin F., The Yoga Sutras of Patanjali (New York: Northpoint Press, 2013)

Burns, Robert Edgar, Complete Poetical Works of Robert Burns (New York: T. Y. Crowell & Co. 1884)

Carrera, Reverend Jaganath, founder of Yoga Life Society (online source)

Clare, John, "I Am!" (source unknown)

Corballis, Michael C., The Lopsided Ape (New York/Oxford: Oxford University Press, 1991)

The Dalai Lama, H.H., The Art of Happiness (New York: Riverhead Books, Penguin Putnam Inc., 1998)

The Dalai Lama, H.H., Consciousness At The Crossroads (Ithaca, N.Y.: Snow Lion Publications, 1999)

The Dalai Lama, H.H.. The Good Heart: A Buddhist Perspective On The Teachings Of Jesus (Boston: Wisdom Publications, 1996)

The Dalai Lama, H.H. Kindness, Clarity, and Insight (Delhi: Motilal Banarsidass Publishers Private Limited, 1997)

The Dalai Lama, H.H. Sleeping, Dreaming and Dying (Boston: Wisdom Publications, 1997)

The Dalai Lama, H.H., "Where Buddhism Meets Neuroscience" (Boulder, CO: Shambhala Publications, 1999)

DeCharms, Christopher, Two Views of Mind (New York: Snow Lion Publications, 1998)

Dechenet, Jean-Marie, Christian Yoga (New York: Harper & Row Publishers, 1960)

Desikachar, T.K.V., The Heart of Yoga (Rochester, VT: Inner Traditions, 1999)

Desikachar, T.K.V., Patanjali's Yogasutras (Madras: Affiliated East-West Press Private Limited, 1987)

Emerson, Ralph Waldo, Journals (October 27, 1831)

Faber, Frederick W., "There's a Wideness in God's Mercy" (source unknown)

Feldman, Christina & Kornfield, Jack, Stories of the Spirit, Stories of the Heart (New York: Harper Collins Publishers, 1991)

Feuerstein, Georg, The Yoga-Sutra Of Patanjali (Rochester, Vermont: Inner Traditions Intl, 1979)

Gibran, Kahlil (source unknown)

H.D. "The Walls Do Not Fall" (New York, Liveright Publishing, 1925)

Helminski, Kabir Edmund . Living Presence (New York: Jeremy P. Tarcher/G.P. Putnam's Sons, 1992)

Hilts, Philip J., Memory's Ghost (New York: Touchstone, 1995)

Jha, Ganganatha, Yoga-Sara-Sangraha of Vijnana- Bhiksu (Delhi, India: Parimal Publications, 1995)

Khan, Pir Hazrat Inayat, "The Teaching of Pir Hazrat Inayat Khan" (Vol. 4, Mental Purification, Section 3 "Unlearning" (online source)

Kraftsow, Gary, American Viniyoga Institute, 1992, 2024

Krishnamacharya, Tirumalai, Yoganjalisaram (Chennai, India: Krishnamacharya Yoga Mandiram, 1976)

Krishnananda, Swami, "The Philosophy of Life, Part One: The Foundations of Philosophy, Chapter 9: Isvara or the Universal Soul (online source)

Lad, Vasant, "Strands of Eternity" (Albuquerque, NM: Ayurvedic Press, 2004)

Leggett, Trevor, The Chapter Of The Self (London and Henley: Routledge & Paul Kegan 1978)

Leggett, Trevor, Sankara on the Yoga Sutras (London: Routledge & Kegan Paul, 1981)

McConkey, James, The Anatomy of Memory (New York: Oxford University Press, l996)

Machado, Antonio, There is no Road (source unknown)

Mechtild of Magdeburg (source unknown)

Nagao, Gadjin M., "Ascent and Descent: Two-Directional Activity in Buddhist Thought" (Presidential Address for The Sixth Conference of The IABS, Tokyo, Japan, September, 1983, online source)

Nischala Joy Devi, The Secret Power of Yoga, A Woman's Guide to the Heart and Spirit of the Yoga Sutras (Louisville, KY: Harmony House 2022)

O'Maolain, Marc extract from "Ishvara Pranidhanam" (Philippines: poemhunter.com)

Osborne, Arthur, "Be Still" Poetry for the Spirit (London Watkins Publishing, 1999)

Pinker, Stephen, How The Mind Works (New York & London: W.W. Norton & Company, 1997)

Prabhupada, Bhaktivedanta Swami , "Srimad-Bhâgavatam" (Delhi: League of Devotees, Vrindaban, 1962)

Prasada, Rama, Patanjali's Yoga Sutras (Munshiram Monoharlal Publishers Pvt., Ltd., 1995)

Rama, Swami, Living With The Himalayan Masters (Honesdale, Pennsylvania; Himalayan International Institute 1978)

Ramachandran, V.S., M.D. and Sandra Blakeslee, Phantoms In The Brain, (New York: William Morrow and Company, Inc., 1998)

Ramana Maharshi, The Spiritual Teaching of Ramana Maharshi (Tiruvanamalai, India: Sri Ramanasramam, 1972)

Rumi, Jalal Al-din,"The Churn", "The Well", "Masnavi","Open the Window" (sources unknown)

Sheng Yen, Chan Master, "Getting the Buddha Mind" (New York: Dharma Drum Publications, 1982)

Tatsuguchi, Wasui, A Study of Shin Buddhism (Honolulu: Shinshu Kyokai Mission Of Hawaii, 1961)

Tola, Fernando, Dragonetti, Carmen, The Yogasutras Of Patanjali [English translation by K. D. Prithipaul] (Delhi: Motilal Barasidass Publishers Pvt. Ltd., 1991)

Wangmo, Geshe Kelsang, The Four Schools of Buddhist Philosophy, Tushita Meditation Centre Course Materials

Whicher, Ian, The Integrity of the Yoga Darsana (New York: State University of New York Press, 1998)

Index Of Sanskrit Terms